Recent Results in Cancer Research 129

K. Höffken (Ed.)

Peptides in Oncology II

Somatostatin Analogues
and Bombesin Antagonists

With 19 Figures and 14 Tables

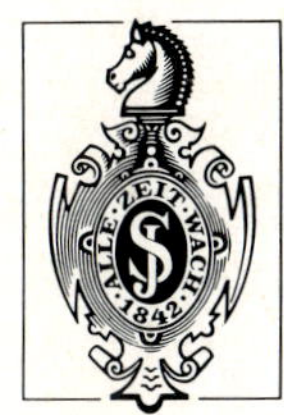

Springer-Verlag
Berlin Heidelberg New York
London Paris Tokyo
Hong Kong Barcelona
Budapest

Prof. Dr. K. Höffken
Klinik für Innere Medizin II: Onkologie – Hämatologie – Endokrinologie – Stoffwechselerkrankungen
Klinikum der Friedrich-Schiller-Universität Jena
Erlanger Allee 101, O-6902 Jena-Lobeda, FRG

ISBN 3-540-56669-4 Springer-Verlag Berlin Heidelberg New York
ISBN 0-387-56669-4 Springer-Verlag New York Berlin Heidelberg

Typesetting, printing, binding: K. Triltsch, Graphischer Betrieb, Würzburg
65/3130-5 4 3 2 1 0 – Printed on acid-free paper

Preface

Controlled and predictable interference with hormonal feedback mechanisms has become a major direction of preclinical and clinical research. There is a steadily increasing number of hormonal peptides detected and characterized that are responsible for endo-, para-, and autocrine cellular actions. Naturally, these peptides have been studied with regard to their cell growth stimulatory action and, in parallel, the respective antagonists are being investigated in terms of their antiproliferative (antineoplastic) function.

Among the numerous peptides of interest in this respect, somatostatin (somatotropin release inhibitory factor) and bombesin antagonizing factors have been the topic of intensive research during recent years. No presentation of the role of peptides in oncology would be complete without a comprehensive treatise of their physiological, preclinical and clinical functions in the context of their antineoplastic mechanism of action.

Somatostatin and its various short- and long-acting analogs have the unique feature of suppressing and inhibiting a wide range of cellular processes including cell proliferation. Receptors for these peptides, which belong in a wider sense to the family of neuropeptides or neurotransmitters, are widely distributed, a feature which is not in keeping with the general view of a growth hormone regulatory system. Thus, these substances are found in the gut in a variety of endocrine and exocrine glands including breast, pancreas, and prostate, and in the nervous system. In addition to playing a physiological role in regulating growth, somatostatin can act directly as an antiproliferative substance, although the mechanism of this action is not yet understood.

In this second volume of peptides in oncology, experts in the field have contributed their knowledge by extensively reviewing the mechanisms of action of somatostatin and its analogs as well as by summarizing the clinical effects of treating patients with pancreatic, breast and small-cell lung cancer. As becomes evident, hopes for this treatment have not yet been fulfilled. As in prostate cancer and other neoplastic diseases known to respond in experimental settings (e.g., chondrosarcoma, bladder cancer, non-small-cell lung cancer, meningiomas, and hepatic metastases from a variety of malignant tumors), present and future clinical investigations of somatostatin treatment alone or in combination with other peptides (e.g., LH-RH) or other cytostatic substances (e.g., cytostatic chemotherapy) have to be elucidated before the exact role of these peptides can be defined.

Somatostatin plays a prominent role in the treatment of neuroendocrine tumors of the gut and in pituitary adenomas. This is excellently reviewed by two authors who have been involved in this field for many years. Clearly, somatostatin and its analogs have gained an established place in the treatment of acromegaly and TSH-producing pituitary adenomas as well as in treating the (endocrine) symptoms of VIPoma, glucagonoma, gastrinoma and the carcinoid syndrome. For a complete picture of the role of somatostatin analogs in oncology, its present status in the treatment of neoplastic pain is discussed in brief. In addition, it is of note that, as was established recently, somatostatin has a prominent effect in severe, treatment-induced (e.g., fluorouracil, total body irradiation for bone marrow transplantation) diarrhea. Somatostastin is also of diagnostic value in detecting intestinal tumors that bear somatostatin receptors using scintigraphy with radiolabeled octreotide.

Bombesin and its related neurotransmitting peptides have been shown to have a wide range of biological and pharmacological actions, including the ability to stimulate the growth of a number of cancer cell lines in vitro. Of most interest in recent years was the discovery of bombesin receptors on small-cell lung cancer cells and the inhibitory effect of bombesin antagonists on such cell lines in vitro. The remarkable body of knowledge now accumulated warranted an indepth description of the classes and function of bombesin receptor antagonists, as well as their role in the treatment of small-cell lung cancer. Here, as with somatostatin, we must await the results of carefully designed clinical trials before we can define the contribution these peptides can make to oncologic treatment.

I trust that this second volume on peptides in oncology will complete the overview of the role of these substances in antineoplastic therapy. It is my firm belief that the ongoing intensive research (e.g., on the correct doses of the peptides or on the choice of the best analog of the numerous substances) will soon provide clinical benefits for patients, beyond the established effects in some entities of pituitary adenomas and neuroendocrine gastrointestinal tumors.

It is my privilege and pleasure to acknowledge the assistance of Mrs. G. Cönenberg and Mrs. G. Stoschek as well as Mrs. S. Benko and Dr. T. Thiekötter for providing their expertise again in the publication of this second volume on peptides in oncology.

Jena, March 1993 K. Höffken

Contents

List of Contributors *

---

* The address of the principal author is given on the first page of each contribution.

[1] Page on which contribution begins.

Somatostatin Analogues

Somatostatin Analogues: Mechanisms of Action

H. Parmar, R.H. Phillips, and S.L. Lightman

Department of Clinical Oncology, Westminster Hospital, Horseferry Road, London SW1 2AP, Great Britain

Introduction

The structure of somatostatin was elucidated by Brazeau et al. in 1973 [13], and scientific work prior to and following the discovery of the structure of the peptide has accelerated at an ever-increasing pace. It has been noted that it can act as an almost universal chalone (a secretion that depresses and inhibits the activity of various intracellular processes). For many years the concept of the existence of an inhibitory hormone for the gastrointestinal tract had been established, and this had been recognised and discussed many times even prior to the discovery of somatostatin. Further research has established that there are several related peptides which make up a family that includes the originally identified 14 amino acid peptide designated somatostatin 14 (SS14) [10], somatostatin 28 (SS28) [34, 41], several species-specific variants, and even larger pro-hormone forms which are secreted in different parts of the body. Therefore, the singular name "somatostatin" is inappropriate, but is widely used and accepted to include all the variants. These peptides are widely distributed beyond the confines of the growth hormone (GH) regulatory system and are found in the gut, in various exocrine and endocrine glands throughout the body, and in most organs. They display highly selective and sometimes specific functions depending upon the anatomical site of localisation and the local physiological environment. For example, SS28 is found among other sites in the central nervous system and has a more potent neuromodulator action than SS14. Furthermore, it has been demonstrated that SS28 has a greater suppressive effect on insulin secretion than SS14 in the pancreas [68]. This differential response seems to depend on the actual size of the peptide, the specific binding of the peptide to the different high-capacity and low-capacity somatostatin receptors discovered, and the latent potency of the peptide.

Somatostatin is also found elsewhere in the nervous system, e.g. in the pituitary gland, the limbic system, and all parts of the brain stem and spinal. cord [3, 47, 48, 54, 55, 78]. In the brain it acts as a neurohormone, neurotransmitter, or neuromodulator. Elsewhere it is found in specific secretory D cells of the gut, pancreas, and salivary glands [6, 7, 31, 38, 70, 81]. In these organs and at other sites it can act as a paracrine secretory factor (local regulator) or as an autocrine secretory factor (self-regulator). The wide-ranging diverse effects of somatostatin in the gastrointestinal system are given in Table 1. These effects occur to a greater or lesser extent in physiological and pathological conditions. A number of these effects can be useful in a wide range of medical conditions including the treatment of cancer patients.

Somatostatin has direct inhibitory effects on insulin, glucagon, secretin, GH, thyroid-stimulating hormone (TSH) and gastrin [1, 8, 104]. It is stimulated by insulin deficiency, glucagon, amino acids, glucose, acetylcholine, vasoactive intestinal polypeptide (VIP), secretin, substance P, gastrin, neurotensin, and prostaglandin E2 [6, 104]. All these hormones are to a greater or lesser extent intricately involved in the regulation of somatostatin at the various anatomical sites. These regulatory processes are further controlled and affected by changes in various intracellular and extracellular processes. For example, in the gastrointestinal system, upon entering the lumen of the gut, somatostatin modifies the secretion of acid and gastrin and has therefore been termed a "lumone" [104].

Table 1. Gastrointestinal effects of somatostatin

1. Inhibits	– Gastrin
	– Pancreozymin
	– Vasoactive intestinal peptide
	– Glucagon
	– Motilin
	– Gastric inhibitory peptide
	– Pancreatic polypeptide
	– Secretin
	– Pepsin, intrinsic factor
2. Inhibits	– Gastric acid secretion
	– Pancreatic bicarbonate
	– Pancreatic enzymes
	– Colonic fluid
	– Bile fluid
3. Inhibits	– Gastric emptying
	– Gallbladder contraction
	– Small intestine contraction
4. Decreases absorption of	– Water
	– Triglycerides
	– Lactose
	– Amino acids
	– Fructose
	– Galactose
	– Xylose
	– Glycerol
	– Glucose
	– Calcium
5. Decreases mesenteric blood flow, increases vascular resistance	

Somatostatin is also found in the kidneys, and may have inhibitory effects on the action of vasopressin and renin [39, 48, 105]. The anatomical distribution of somatostatin and its physiology, biochemistry, and pharmacological effects have been reviewed extensively in recently published articles [6, 36, 73, 102–104]. It is beyond the scope of this chapter to cover these aspects in detail, but the reader is referred to these articles for comprehensive coverage of such details.

One of the many important functions of somatostatin, apart from the hormonal and other effects mentioned above, is to act as a natural growth inhibitor with antiproliferative properties. Somatostatin has been shown to have inhibitory effects on numerous cellular processes including cell replication [130]. These effects are of considerable importance in oncology where there is a constant need to develop new anticancer agents with high therapeutic efficacy and low toxicity, both in curative and palliative treatment [28, 61]. This chapter will now concentrate specifically on the general mechanisms of action, the rationale and the present and future potential applications of these actions on different tumours. The recent development of long-acting somatostatin analogues with more prolonged and enhanced pharmacological activity will be discussed with reference to the treatment of a wide range of different cancers.

Somatostatin Analogues

The comparative amino acid sequences of somatostatin and some of the commercially developed analogues is given in Fig. 1. The natural peptide somatostatin has a plasma half-life of about 3 min, since it is rapidly broken down by digestive enzymes including peptidase. Therapeutic application of the native hormone has, therefore, been limited, since prolonged continuous intravenous treatment is necessary to produce a therapeutic effect. Furthermore, subsequent immediate rebound of the therapeutic effect has been noted following withdrawal of somatostatin, and this is associated with a rapid rise in target hormones [61]. This rebound effect is, therefore, troublesome, particularly in situations where prolonged continuous activity is absolutely essential, and the phenomenon should be avoided as much as possible in cancer patients, since tumour growth should not be allowed if at all possible. It is, therefore, clear, that there is an absolute need for longer acting analogues, and with this in mind a number of commercial peptides have come to the clinic and are being developed for many indications.

It is clear from the amino acid sequence of somatostatin shown in Fig. 1 that a large number of analogues can be produced by amino acid substitution at various sites along the peptide chain [22]. It has been found that a sequence of only eight amino acids is now recognised as necessary to simulate and enhance the actions of SS14, although smaller peptides (including a tetrapeptide) have also been synthesised and shown to have some activity. D-Amino acid substitutions greatly enhance the activity of such analogues and thereby alter differ-

```
S-----------------------------------S
|                                   |
Ala-Gly-Cys-Lys-Asn-Phe-Phe-Trp-Lys-Thr-Phe-Thr-Ser-Cys-OH
```

Somatostatin 14

```
      S-----------------S
      |                 |
D-Phe-Cys-Phe-D-Trp-Lys-Thr-Cys-Thr(ol)
```

SMS 201-995

```
      S-----------------S
      |                 |
D-Phe-Cys-Tyr-D-Trp-Lys-Val-Cys-Trp-NH2
```

RC-160

```
        S-----------------S
        |                 |
D-βNal-Cys-Tyr-D-Trp-Lys-Val-Cys-Thr-NH2
```

BIM 23014

Fig. 1. Amino acid sequences of somatostatin 14, SMS 201-995, RC-160, and BIM-23014 for comparison

ent receptor-binding specificity, activity, and site of action. A prolonged plasma half-life can also be produced, depending on which of the amino acids are substituted. Apart from the eight amino acids, the sulphide bridge seems to be an essential part of the molecule for therapeutic activity. This is probably also the essential part of the molecule for receptor-binding activity. The amino acid sequence of the three most widely tested octapeptide analogues of somatostatin are also shown in Fig. 1.

These superanalogues or agonists are relatively resistant to proteolytic enzymes mainly due to the substituted D-amino acids, and therefore have longer half-lives of up to several hours. They can thus be selected for specific actions and target sites, which means that a large number of clinical applications become more feasible. Furthermore, some of these analogues do not seem to have the immediate "rebound" effect seen with somatostatin [27, 61, 69] as one would expect, since these analogues have longer plasma half-lives and the therapeutic effect takes longer to wear off. Before we discuss the exact general and specific mechanisms of action of such analogues at each tumor site, we need to understand the basic pharmacological and hormonal effects. These will be discussed prior to the antiproliferative effects, which will then be discussed separately in general and subsequently applied briefly to some tumour sites which have already been shown to respond to such therapy; potential future areas of research in other tumours will also be discussed.

Pharmacological and Hormonal Effects

A number of pharmacological studies of the different somatostatin analogues have been reported and published [79]. Essentially, Sandostatin, an octapeptide (SMS 201-995; Sandoz, Basel, Switzerland), was the first commercially available analogue to be extensively studied in a wide range of human tumours. Pharmacological studies have shown it to be 45 times more potent than the natural somatostatin in releasing GH and 11 times more potent in the inhibition of glucagon. It is 1.3 times more active in the inhibition of insulin secretion than natural somatostatin, SS14 [58]. Sandostatin needs to be given by subcutaneous injection three to four times a day and has an elimination half-life of 113 min [69]. The plasma half-life is about 40% – 50% shorter when given by i.v. infusion. A slow-release formulation of sandostatin which may last 1 – 4 weeks depending upon dose and indication is undergoing pharmacological testing in several centres around the world.

Oral preparations of somatostatin analogues have also been tested, and therapeutic activity has been demonstrated [133] but very large dosages need to be given (4 – 8 mg, three times a day). The bioavailability is 40 – 80 times less than the equivalent therapeutic subcutaneous dose. In view of these factors and further cost considerations, this is not a practicable way of delivering the drug to the target sites, and this route of administration has now been abandoned by most investigators.

Somatuline, also an octapeptide (BIM-23014; Ipsen Biotech, Paris, France), was selected for study by our group from many other octapeptide analogues of the natural 14 amino acid somatostatin. The structural chemical formula of somatuline is given in Fig. 1. It was chosen with the intention of finding an analogue with little effect on insulin and glucagon secretion but a more profound effect on GH and GH dependent growth factors such as insulin-like growth factor (IGF-I), also called somatomedin C. Somatuline has been shown to have more selective peripheral actions rather than the central actions some other somatostatin analogues have. It also has a prolonged duration of action, with plasma activity lasting for several hours rather than minutes. Its half-life has been calculated to be approximately 80 – 90 min.

Somatuline is a white odourless powder that is soluble in water, has a molecular formula of C54H69N11O10S2 and with a molecular weight of 1096.34. It has been tested and can be administered by several different routes, namely by intravenous infusion (either as a bolus or a slow infusion over many hours or days), by subcutaneous bolus injection, or by continuous subcutaneous infusion using any standard syringe driver. Recently a slow-release preparation has been developed in a microencapsulated formulation bound in a matrix of polylactide-glycolide microspheres which is administered by deep intramuscular injection. The polymer is completely biodegradable and biocompatible and contains 30 mg of BIM-23014, which is administered at 1 – 2 weekly intervals, depending upon the clinical indications. Longer acting formulations, lasting up to 4 weeks are also undergoing pharmacological testing.

The process to produce a slow-release formulation for all the analogues has been difficult and is partly marred by the high doses of drug required to be released into the circulation to maintain the tissue levels of the analogues at sufficiently high level to suppress GH. Wide fluctuations in plasma levels from these slow release formulations make it difficult to maintain constant suppressed levels of GH. Therefore it is not surprising that GH escape occurs in some patients at certain dosages. This was our experience when we treated 36 patients with prostate cancer and compared the effect of the slow-release formulation with the subcutaneous infusion pump [89, 90]. However, IGF-I suppression was achieved in a large proportion of patients in both groups, despite the failure of full suppression of GH at the low dosages used (<1.5 mg per day). This phenomenon is entirely due to the competitive nature of GH inhibition by all analogues. There seems to be a certain absolute requirement in the plasma level of these analogues to achieve continuous GH suppression. Down-regulation of the somatostatin receptor does not seem to occur, even on prolonged continuous administration, unlike the effect of luteinizing hormone-releasing hormone (LHRH) agonists on their receptors [83–87]. This, therefore, explains the difficulty in producing good slow-release formulations of such analogues. New and innovative methods of delivery are needed, however, and some of these are currently being tested for all the different analogues to make administration more convenient for patients.

As far as the hormonal effects are concerned, somatuline's rate of inhibition of gastric acid secretion is 39%, whilst other analogues in the same series have a more powerful inhibitory effect of up to 89% (Table 2). Conversely, there is some evidence that the analogues that have maximal effects on gastric acid secretion have less significant effects on GH secretion, and vice versa. This differential response can be used to maximise clinical benefit and minimise adverse physiological effects, which becomes a significant advantage in the particular potential clinical applications envisaged for that particular analogue. This point is stressed to indicate that not all analogues of somatostatin have the same physiological and pharmacological effects, and the doses of the various analogues required to produce the same effect may be very different. However, because of commercial interests and the costs associated with the

Table 2. Inhibition rate of gastric acid and growth hormone by different somatostatin analogues

Analogue	Inhibition of gastric acid (%)	Inhibition of growth hormone (%)
BIM-23014	39.7	95.7
BIM-23025	38.0	93.3
BIM-23027	74.9	85.1
BIM-23023	80.2	74.8
BIM-23022	88.8	–
BIM-23026	89.5	77.9

development of such drugs, only a limited number of analogues can be developed for clinical use. It is quite conceivable that some extremely important analogues with very special enhanced activity in some particular effect may never be developed because of the cost involved.

The physiological and hormonal effects of somatuline in animal studies will be summarised briefly. In rats, somatuline caused 96% inhibition of GH releasing factor (GRF; growth hormone releasing hormone, GHRH) stimulation of GH release at a dose of 200 μg/kg, and at a dose of 100 μg/kg it caused 84% inhibition. In cynomolgus monkeys, 250 μg of somatuline administered subcutaneously suppressed the GH peaks induced by arginin 1 h and 4 h after treatment [88].

In patients with acromegaly, administration of 500 μg BIM-23014 subcutaneously typically leads to a rapid rise in plasma levels of the drug, with an almost immediate suppression of GH which is maintained for about 6 h after a single injection. The plasma half-life of somatuline in this experiment was determined to be approximately 90 min [88].

When up to 500 μg/day was administered subcutaneously in two daily doses, BIM-23014 failed to fully suppress arginine-stimulated GH secretion in five patients with pancreatic cancer, as one would expect from the short half-life of all such analogues. At higher dosages (3 mg or more given by 24-h subcutaneous infusion), however, it is very effective in suppressing GH release: all five patients treated with the slow-release formulation of somatuline achieved suppression of hGHRH stimulation of IGF-I, and this was maintained for up to 10 days following each injection, despite the fact that the GH levels were not suppressed in all patients. Higher dosages of up to 12 mg/day by continuous subcutaneous infusion are now being evaluated in similar patients with pancreatic cancer, and as expected, the higher doses are much more effective in suppressing GH and IGF-I.

In acute toxicity studies, a dose of somatuline up to 100 times greater than the initial human therapeutic dose (1.5 mg/day) given subcutaneously or intravenously failed to produce any significant toxicity, and the LD_{50} for rats or mice could not be determined. Toxicity studies conducted for over 2 years in rats and dogs have failed to demonstrate any significant toxicity, and no mutagenic effects have been observed. The incidence of side effects is low, and they tend to be generally mild and/or transient and never require interruption of treatment. With subcutaneous injections, slight pain and redness have been observed in approximately 8% of patients. Mild diarrhoea, abdominal pain, and cramps have been reported in volunteers given doses of up to 2–4 mg in 24 h. In insulin-controlled diabetics, a 10%–20% reduction of insulin is sometimes necessary but severe hypoglycaemia has not been a problem; this should, however, be monitored with routine glucose levels.

With the sustained-release formulation, mild to moderate pain occurs around the injection site in approximately 10% of patients. This is usually transient and subsides after a few minutes to a few hours. Patients on prolonged continuous administration of these analogues are at risk of developing gall stones; this may occur in up to 15%–20% of patients treated with such analogues for more than 6 months. A routine ultrasound scan of the upper abdomen is recommended here.

Antiproliferative Effects

The mechanism of action of somatostatin is not well understood despite the extensive research which has been carried out over the past 20 years. Specifically binding somatostatin receptors have been demonstrated in the central nervous system and in several peripheral organs [44, 62, 95]. The minimal structure of the active receptor(s) has been identified, and active high-capacity and low-capacity receptors have been found in different organs, including the brain, gastrointestinal system, and certain tumours. Somatostatin receptors have been found in human meningioma, and breast and carcinoid tumours [108, 109], and also on hormone-responsive prostate Dunning R3327H tumours [51] in rats. Thus, these receptors are found in normal, benign and malignant tissues. Their biological function is unclear, although interaction with such receptors may comprise one of the mechanisms by which somatostatin analogues exert a general antiproliferative effect. Binding affinities of SS14, SS28 and somatostatin analogues show different organ specificities, implying the existence of several different receptor subtypes [62] and perhaps different levels of activity of the different analogues modulated through these receptors.

GH has been implicated as one of a number of factors in tumour proliferation. Physiologically, GH secretion is regulated by the interaction of several important factors. It is stimulated by hypothalamic GHRH and inhibited by the effects of somatostatin. Superimposed on this system is a feedback loop involving both GH and the growth factors called, somatomedins (e.g. IGF-I). The somatomedins are produced by the liver under the influence of GH. IGF-I has a direct negative feedback on the pituitary gland by blocking the action of GHRH.

The role of GH on the regulation of GHRH is not yet fully worked out. It has been shown that one of the functions of GH is to stimulate cellular differentiation directly and through local production of growth factors [24, 26, 45, 81, 98, 138]. All the growth factors including IGF-I, epidermal growth factor (EGF), platelet-derived growth factor (PDGF), fibroblast growth factor (FGF), transforming growth factor (TGF and TGF-β), bombesin and probably other as yet undiscovered growth factors are intricately involved in the proliferation of normal, benign, and malignant cells [5, 26, 42, 45, 49, 119, 122, 126, 131]. Somatostatin has also been shown to have inhibitory effects on these growth factors and in some cases reduces the levels, either by a direct effect on the growth factors or through the reduction of GH [52, 128]. These effects can be used to therapeutic advantage in a wide range of tumours and will be discussed specifically later with the individual tumour subtypes.

Somatostatin and somatostatin analogues also have other specific direct inhibitory effects on cell proliferation [30, 99, 128]. It has been shown that somatostatin inhibits rapid centrosomal separation and cell proliferation induced by EGF [70]. In dividing cells, centrosomal separation is a biological marker of the G_1 phase in the cycling cell, and this effect of somatostatin is associated with suppression of DNA synthesis and suppression of cell replication. The exact mechanism by which somatostatin inhibits centrosomal separation is not clear, but it may involve interference with microfilaments, stabilisation of microtubules, and/or inhibition or changes in intracellular calcium signals [70]. These specific actions need to be further elucidated, and several interventional strategies are under investigation. Some of these effects on cell replication are also known to occur with certain cytotoxic agents, and novel new chemotherapy regimes need to be devised in combination with such analogues in all stages of cancer. Some of these combination regimes may need to be used early and in the adjuvant setting in the treatment of such cancers in order to maximise the benefits of such antiproliferatives. The interaction of Levimasole and 5-fluorouracil (5-FU) in large-bowel cancer is one good example where the appropriate use of a combination of two relatively inactive agents in Dukes stage C carcinoma have been shown to improve survival in a significant proportion of patients. Similar therapeutic strategies need to be devised for somatostatin analogues in combination with chemotherapy in a wide range of tumours if we are to see survival benefits due to such peptides.

Somatostatin has other specific and nonspecific modulatory effects on the immune system which may be beneficial in anticancer therapy [88]. Somatostatin analogues have been shown to stimulate the function of the reticuloendothelial system in the rat [9]. This increase in immune function may by very relevant in the adjuvant setting for the treatment of cancer when only small-volume microscopic disease may still be present in patients treated by surgery [91]. In this setting, it is possible for a small change in the immune function to lead to a large overall benefit. In one controlled study, treatment with the somatostatin analogue Sandostatin significantly inhibited the growth and development of hepatic metastases induced in rats [82]. It is not known whether this effect was associated with stimulation of the immune system, with a direct inhibitory effect on tumour growth, or with the prevention of metastases by preventing angiogenesis or some other mechanism. Any or all of these mechanisms may be operative in this situation. Such a response could certainly be of potential benefit in several human tumours commonly associated with hepatic metastases following definitive primary surgical treatment, such as in carcinomas of the colon, breast, and lung. Clearly a randomised trial on the same lines as the Levimasole study in colon cancer is perhaps necessary in humans to evaluate this effect. This would, of course, become feasible with the development of slow-release formulations lasting for at least 1 week.

Other antiproliferative effects of somatostatin have also been shown. Somatostatin stimulates dephosphorylation of membrane receptors and proteins which are usually activated and promoted by phosphorylation mediated through EGF [46]. Following binding of EGF to its receptor, there is activation of protein kinase C and phosphorylation of membrane receptors, which is a key step in cellular proliferation [135]. This may be one mechanism by which SS14 and somatostatin analogues exert inhibitory effects on EGF and other growth factors and receptors.

It has been postulated that normal cellular proliferation involves both autocrine and paracrine stimulatory phenomena [127]. With such a hypothesis, normal control of growth involves the differential response to different tonic concentrations of several growth-regulatory hormones or factors at once. If this is the case, then minor changes in the relative concentrations of these different regulators might induce small or dramatic changes in cell morphology, physiology, and biochemistry, and in the growth of such cells.

The findings that IGFs may act by paracrine or autocrine mechanisms [120] and that concentrations of IGF-I are GH dependent [24] would seem to suggest that certain cancers should be responsive to somatostatin or its analogues. However, since the production of autocrine growth factors may be a mechanism for escape from normal physiological control, there may be little relationship between the doses required for inhibiting normal physiological activity and that required for "direct" antitumour effects. This point is emphasised since the apparent limited activity that has been observed in some experimental tumour systems appears to be dose related [11]. The doses required for such activity in human tumours may be far in excess of that routinely prescribed up to now. Our experience in human tumours is in keeping with these observations. Low or no responses were seen at lower dosages but higher responses have been observed at higher dosages (unpublished data).

Furthermore, the tumour growth inhibitory effects obtained with antiproliferatives are evolving more slowly in contrast to the dramatic oncolytic effects that are induced with cytotoxic chemotherapeutic agents: this observation suggests that early stabilisation of disease is a positive therapeutic response and one which may lead to tumour regression after some indeterminate time. Our clinical experience in some patients with prostate cancer is in keeping with these observations. Initial stabilization after 3 months was followed by partial remission on continued treatment at 6–12 months.

Therefore, the importance of attaining and maintaining adequate high concentrations of somatostatin analogues at the site of a proliferating cell population cannot be overemphasised, since it is possible that in some instances locally produced somatomedins may bind immediately to receptor sites, or that locally produced binding proteins [20, 29] may interfere with somatostatin binding to its target cell. This may be an important factor in certain tumours. Adequately high concentrations of somatostatin analogues are, therefore, essential for a therapeutic effect. Local effects of somatostatin analogues need further investigation and intradermal infiltration needs to be evaluated for some tumours such as acquired immunodeficiency syndrome (AIDS)-related Kaposi sarcoma and malignant melanoma.

Acromegaly and Other Pituitary Tumours

Acromegaly and other pituitary tumours are benign in nature and symptoms are caused by local expansion of the tumour into vital structures and the secondary effects of this, associated with the production of abnormal amounts of specific hormones. Responses to somatostatin analogues [25, 57, 140] in patients with acromegaly, GH/prolactin-secreting adenomas and TSH-secreting pituitary tumours are, therefore, expected and have been reported. Pituitary tumours associated with acromegaly may be large, and if they fail to respond or relapse after surgical and radiation therapy, medical treatment is indicated for progressive clinical symptoms and signs. Bromocriptine is the usual first-line therapy recommended in this situation, but it rarely produces sufficient suppression of GH [60]. Somatostatin analogues are more effective in GH suppression and better tolerated in acromegalic patients. Several small clinical studies have been published which demonstrate considerable therapeutic efficacy in acromegalic patients [14, 15, 18, 47, 58, 59, 127]. Long-term follow-up of these patients has shown virtual disappearance of the clinical signs and symptoms of this disease, and near normalization of laboratory tests. Tumour shrinkage (on computed tomography scan) has also been reported [14, 127]. Therefore, formulations of somatostatin analogues can now be considered as important medical adjuncts in the treatment of acromegaly. They can be used before and following definitive surgery and/or radiotherapy and subsequently following relapse from primary treatment.

Gastrointestinal Peptide-Secreting Tumours

All the various tumours in the group of gastrointestinal peptide-secreting tumours are rare and produce specific syndromes related to the predominant peptide secreted by the tumour. They all tend to arise from the amine precursor uptake and decarboxylation (APUD) cells and have a common embryological origin. Most of these tumours have the capacity to produce a large number of peptides and related clinical syndromes [136]. The majority of the tumours arise from the pancreatic islet cells and tend to follow a relatively benign course, although all have the capacity for metastatic spread and may lead to early death. Somatostatin analogues have been used in a range of these gut and pancreatic peptide-secreting tumours [65, 137]. In insulinomas, for example, somatostatin analogues have been used to relieve symptoms; this has been tested, and clinical benefit reported [37], which is usually of a symptomatic nature, although tumour regression should be an aim. Larger doses than previously used should be tried to bring about a regression. Similar hormone inhibitory principles apply to glucagonoma, which are predominantly malignant but slow growing and with a long history of symptoms related to mild diabetes mellitus, normochromic normocytic anaemia, deep vein thrombosis and pulmonary embolism, diarrhoea and a skin rash. Such patients have been reported to respond symptomatically to somatostatin analogue therapy [16, 17]. Objective evidence of tumour shrinkage has also been reported in such studies following treatment with the somatostatin analogue Sandostatin.

VIP-secreting tumours (also called Verner Morrison syndrome) are predominantly malignant and pancreatic in origin. They are associated with elevated VIP levels, watery diarrhoea, hypokalaemia, achlorhydria, abdominal pain, and weight loss. Somatostatin inhibitis VIP activity and various therapeutic clinical studies have been undertaken. Dramatic clinical benefit with improvement in symptoms and weight gain has been reported and life-threatening diarrhoea has been controlled [19, 53, 71, 106, 134]. Objective tumour shrinkage has also been reported, indicating an important role for somatostatin analogues in such patients [19, 53].

Gastrinomas (also called Zollinger-Ellison syndrome) have a positive family history of other endocrinopathies and are usually present with multiple malignant primary tumours. These patients have intractable peptic ulceration extending from the stomach into the duodenum and jejunum, with or without chronic diarrhoea and steatorrhoea, and elevated levels of plasma gastrin. Somatostatin analogues can be used to these tumours, and various analogues have been tested for their efficacy in suppressing gastrin and gastric acid secretion. Small clinical studies have confirmed the therapeutic benefit of somatostatin analogue treatment of Zollinger-Ellison syndrome [12, 16, 17, 32, 33], and tumour regression has also been reported [115].

Pancreatic polypeptide-secreting and neurotensin-secreting tumours may also respond to somatostatin analogues, but such pure secreting tumours are very rare. GRF-producing tumours have also been reported to respond to these agents [129]. In all such tumours, somatostatin analogues can be used to complement existing therapy, which may or may not be completely effective or curative. Palliation and symptomatic benefits are certainly worthwhile gains in such patients.

Carcinoid Syndrome

Carcinoid syndrome is a rare disorder usually associated with carcinoid tumours of the small bowel which have metastasized to the liver. Occasionally the syndrome occurs with secondaries arising from primary carcinoid tumours of the lung, stomach, and pancreas. Clinically the syndrome usually presents with episodic flushing, diarrhoea and right-sided valvular heart disease in the late stages. Biochemically there is an elevated level of serotonin in plasma and of 5-hydroxyindoleacetic acid (5-HIAA) in the 24-h urinary collection.

Various factors have been described to indicate that this tumour may be responsive to somatostatin analogues. Carcinoid tumours have been shown to have a high density of somatostatin receptors [109]. Further it has been demonstrated that somatostatin can block the carcinoid flush induced by pentagastrin and reduce the circulating levels of serotonin and urinary 5-HIAA levels. Therefore, several clinical studies have been completed, and useful symptomatic and objective tumour regression has been reported [16, 17, 23, 31, 56, 121], with significant falls in 5-HIAA levels. These responses have been maintained for several years in some patients.

Our experience with BIM-23014 has been similar, but was gained in a small group of 19 patients [14]. Somatostatin analogues, therefore, represent an important advance in the management of patients with carcinoid syndrome and should be considered as first-line treatment, perhaps in combination with other therapies in view of the lack of side effects of such analogues. Chemotherapy is usually no more effective than such analogues, but its side effect tend to be greater.

Small-Cell Lung Cancer

Small-cell lung cancer comprises 30% of the total of lung cancers which are the commonest cause of cancer deaths in men. Human small-cell lung cancer exhibits various neuroendocrine features and may have the same embryological origins as APUD cells. Half of the patients with small-cell lung cancer have widespread metastases at the time of diagnosis, and standard first-line treatment consists of combination chemotherapy. Response rates as high as 80% have been reported [21, 96], but despite these results relapse is frequent and survival beyond 2 years is only 5% [2, 34].

EGF receptors have been clearly demonstrated in human lung cancer cell lines [43, 108, 116], and IGF-I has been shown to be a powerful mitogen for small-cell lung cancer [67]. Tumour DNA ploidy has also once again been shown to be an important prognostic determinant [139]. High-affinity somatostatin receptors have been demonstrated in NCI-H69 human lung cancer cell lines [124]. Furthermore, bombesin, a powerful growth factor for human small-cell lung cancer cell lines [135], plays an important role in the growth of this cancer. The effects of bombesin are mediated through protein kinase C and the EGF receptor, and growth regulation of small-cell lung cancer is partly controlled by this mechanism [135]. Since somatostatin interferes with the action of EGF receptors and may inhibit growth through this mechanism, it is a logical step to try and inhibit this tumour type. In vitro and in vivo inhibition of human small-cell lung cancer has been demonstrated by the somatostatin analogue BIM-23014 [123]. Clinical studies using this slow-release analogue are in progress. It is hoped that this nontoxic agent will acquire a useful place in the management of some patients with small-cell lung cancer.

Pancreatic Cancer

New cases of pancreatic cancer diagnosed every year represent over 5% of all cancers and 90% of them arise from the exocrine glands of the pancreas. Exocrine pancreatic cancer is largely resistant to chemotherapy and radiotherapy, and the prognosis is very poor. Theve et al. have reported a median survival of only 10 weeks following diagnosis [125].

The aetiology of this cancer is unknown, although various factors have been implicated. Secretin, cholecystokinin (CCK), GH, and other gastrointestinal peptides produce hyperplasia, hypertrophy, and stimulation of ductal pancreatic adenocarcinoma cell lines [28, 50, 63, 97]. Oestrogen [4] and androgen receptors have been demonstrated in some pancreatic cancers and antioestrogen and LHRH-agonist treatments have been reported to be beneficial in a few patients [40]. Since somatostatin has its major effects on the hormones and secretions of the pancreas including secretin, CCK, GH, and other growth factors and in view of the very poor prognosis and the lack of effective treatment, somatostatin analogues have been proposed as a therapeutic option for pancreatic cancer on the basis of several experimental findings [40, 66]. Production and expression of TGF has been demonstrated by human pancreatic cancer cells [117]. TGF is 10–100 times more potent than EGF in its effect on cellular proliferation and acts through the EGF receptor. EGF receptor overexpression has also been clearly demonstrated in human pancreatic cancer cell lines. Here TGF binds to the EGF receptor and acts as a superagonist autocrine growth regulator [126].

The actions of TGF have, therefore, been strongly implicated in the growth of pancreatic cancer cells and somatostatin has been shown to interfere with the activity of EGF and EGF receptors. In other studies, somatostatin has been shown to stimulate dephosphorylation of membrane receptors which have an antiproliferative effect in MIA PaCa-2 cell lines [46]. Further, pancreatic cancer tumour models have been reported to respond to somatostatin analogues [92, 101]. Tumour shrinkage and reduction in growth rates have been demonstrated.

Clinical studies are in progress in patients with pancreatic cancer, and results are awaited with adequate follow-up to assess the place of these analogues. Our data using a dosage of up to 1.5 mg BIM-23014 per day subcutaneously have failed to demonstrate any tumour regression in 15 patients. Three patients stabilised for a few months, but later developed progressive disease and died from it. However, we have demonstrated that this dose was not effective in fully suppressing GH, and further studies are in progress using much higher dosages up to 12 mg/day. We have demonstrated a significant fall in the most specific pancreatic cancer tumour marker, CA 19-9, in two of five patients treated at a higher dosage of 6 mg/day. Good symptomatic improvement in these patients has also been shown, and they continue on therapy at present. Increasing and higher doses are at present under investigation.

Prostate Cancer

Patients with prostatic cancer usually respond to hormonal manipulation involving androgen deprivation using either medical or surgical castration [83, 85]. After a variable period of response, most patients with advanced metastatic prostatic cancer develop progressive disease and eventually die from their cancer. Various prognostic factors have been implicated in determining the eventual outcome of this disease. High prolactin levels have been correlated with a poor prognosis [77], and raised GH levels have been linked to an increased metastatic potential of prostatic cancer. Somatostatin suppresses the levels of prolactin and GH, and this may be beneficial in this tumour. EGF receptors have been identified in prostatic cancer [132], and tumour DNA ploidy has been shown to be an important prognostic factor. Aneuploid tumours have been shown to have a worse prognosis. Various growth factors (including FGF and EGF) have been identified in the control of normal and malignant prostate tissues [72, 76, 93, 94, 118]. Somatostatin inhibits the effects of some of these growth factors and has direct effects on DNA synthesis and cell replication. Therefore, aneuploid tumours would be expected to respond to these analogues. This prognostic factor needs to be evaluated in a clinical study.

As mentioned previously, somatostatin receptors have also been demonstrated in the Dunning R3327H rat prostate adenocarcinoma model [51], and tumour growth inhibition with somatostatin analogues has been confirmed [80]. The effect of castration in slowing tumour growth was identical to that of BIM-23014 in this experiment. There were no significant changes seen in the testes of the rats treated with somatostatin analogue. This response was not mediated through a reduction in testosterone, which was not suppressed. The exact mechanism of action of these analogues in prostatic cancer remains to be elucidated, but any number of all of the above-mentioned mechanisms may be responsible.

Clinical studies have commenced in patients with prostatic cancer, and early results are encouraging, although further data in a large number of patients will be required. We have treated 36 patients with advanced metastatic prostate cancer who relapsed after conventional therapy with various dosages (up to 6 mg/day) of the somatostatin analogue somatuline. Three patients have achieved a true partial remission, and seven patients have had stable disease for over 6 months [89, 90]. Further it has been suggested that somatostatin analogues should be used as adjuncts to the LHRH agonists in the initial treatment of prostatic cancer [113]. Randomised trials against standard therapy (singly or in combination) will be necessary to evaluate the role of this new agent in prostatic cancer.

Breast Cancer

Breast cancer is the commonest malignancy to affect women, and various prognostic factors have been implicated in its clinical progression. High levels of oestrogen and progesterone receptors on breast tumours have been shown to improve prognosis, while increased prolactin levels in the plasma have been associated with a poorer prognosis and increased metastatic potential [35]. Somatostatin and somatostatin analogues inhibit prolactin release, and this effect may, therefore, be of benefit in the management of the disease. Certainly bromocriptine, an agent which decreases prolactin release, has been suggested and tried as adjuvant treatment [35]. The benefits of such an approach have not yet been fully evaluated.

The detection of EGF receptors has been implicated in a poorer prognosis and is a powerful predictor of early recurrence and death from breast cancer [111]. Tumour DNA ploidy has been shown to be an important prognostic factor in breast cancer [75], whereby aneuploid tumours have a poorer prognosis than diploid tumours. Breast cancer cells [64] have been shown to secrete IGF-I, a polypeptide with confirmed mitogenic activity and autocrine growth factor properties and which has been implicated in the regulation of the growth of breast cancer cells. Somatostatin inhibits the action of certain growth factors including IGF and EGF either directly or indirectly through suppression of GH. The direct inhibitory effects of somatostatin on cellular proliferation processes including DNA synthesis and centrosomal cell separation may be of considerable interest in this tumour. Somatostatin receptors have been identified in breast cancer cells, and somatostatin analogues have been demonstrated to have a direct delaying effect on the growth of human breast cancer cell lines [112, 114]. Rat mammary carcinoma regression has been reported following suppression of GH and prolactin [105, 110]. Since this same effect can be achieved with somatostatin analogues, clinical studies are necessary. In experimental studies, BIM-23014 had a significant ($p<0.001$) inhibitory effect on tumour growth in studies in vivo using transplanted breast cancer cell lines [88]. Using the subrenal capsular assay, BIM-23014 was shown to be effective in a dose-dependent manner in reducing the growth rate of the MCF-7 human breast cancer cell line in rodents. At a dose of 50 μg/kg per day subcutaneously BIM-23014 was significantly superior to ovariectomy.

Oestrogen dependency does not appear to be a prerequisite for the breast tumour inhibitory activity of BIM-23014 [88]. In a similar study, the response of an oestrogen-insensitive rat mammary adenocarcinoma to the somatostatin analogue was evaluated in ovariectomised animals. This tumour was derived from an oestrogen responsive MT/W9a tumour that was escaping castration effects.

Early clinical studies in patients with relapsed breast cancer treated with the somatostatin analogue BIM-23014 are promising. Further clinical studies are in progress at higher dosages and in earlier stages.

Other Tumours

It has been suggested that various hormonal agents may play an important role in the growth and differentiation of normal and malignant cartilage tissue. GH, somatomedins, insulin and glucocorticosteroids stimulate the growth of normal cartilage and the malignant chondrocytes from chondrosarcomas [74]. IGF-I is produced in proliferating chondrocytes and plays an important role as an autocrine or paracrine factor in the growth regulation of these cells [81]. Somatostatin analogues can, therefore, be expected to have an inhibitory effect on the growth of these tumours, and this has been confirmed in experimental studies where chondrosarcomas were transplanted into rats [100, 107]. Clinical studies are now necessary in patients with chondrosarcomas which have relapsed following conventional therapy.

Somatostatin analogues may also be considered for studies in several other human cancers where conventional treatment is unsatisfactory. Bladder cancer exhibits a high expression of EGF receptors which represent a significant prognostic factor. The currently used chemotherapy regime for this cancer, although it is improving, is not very effective and tends to be rather toxic. Non-small-cell lung cancer remains relatively resistant to chemotherapy, and the only effective treatment available for selected patients are radical surgery and radiotherapy. The use of somatostatin analogues should be investigated here. Meningioma have a high concentration of somatostatin receptors, and this is one good reason for trying somatostatin analogues in patients who have relapsed after primary treatment with surgery and/or radiotherapy. The possibility of using these analogues in preventing hepatic metastasis has already been discussed, and such an approach in large-bowel cancer would have some rationale and validity.

Conclusions

With continuing research and our deeper understanding of the physiology, biochemistry, and pharmacological actions of somatostatin analogues and with an ever-expanding stock of knowledge of tumour molecular biology, growth control, and pathogenesis, many other tumours may become candidates for clinical trials with somatostatin analogues. Somatostatin analogues are not only research tools, but are being demonstrated to be therapeutic agents with wide clinical application. Significant activity already has been demonstrated for these analogues with minimal side effects [19, 53, 56, 90]. It is clear that somatostatin analogues have a remarkable number and variety of actions in different parts of the body. In addition to the well-defined hormonal effects, these agents have powerful actions on cell differentiation and division. The wider application of these agents in oncology are only now being appreciated. Further research with somatostatin analogues and other peptides will help to unravel the complex process of inhibiting the cellular proliferation so characteristic of cancer. The dawn of a new therapeutic modality for the treatment of cancer is being opened up by such peptides. We can look forward optimistically to other similar agents which will arrive from the research being carried out in molecular biology and from the human genome project which remains an urgent priority for the next decade.

References

1. Adrian TE, Barnes AJ, Long RG, O'Shaughnessy DJ, Brown MR, Rivier J, Vale W, Blackburn AM, Bloom SR (19891) The effect of somatostatin analogs on secretion of growth, pancreatic and gastrointestinal hormones in man. J Clin Endocrinol Metab 53:675–681
2. Aisner J, Alberto P, Bitran J, Comis R, Daniels J, Hansen H, Ikegami H, Smyth J (1983) Role of chemotherapy in SCLC – a consensus report of the International Association for Study of Lung Cancer Workshop. Cancer Treat Rep 67:37–40
3. Alpert LC, Brawer JR, Patel YC, Reichlin S (1976) Somatostatinergic neurons in anterior hypothalamus: immunohistochemical localisation. Endocrinology 98:255–258

4. Andren-Sandberg A (1986) Estrogens and pancreatic cancer: some recent aspects. Scand J Gastroenterol 21:129–133
5. Antoniades HN, Pantazis P, Graves DT, Owen AJ, Tempst P (1985) Platelet-derived growth factor: a link to malignant transformation. In: Feramisco J et al. (eds) Cancer cells three: growth factors and transformation. Cold Spring Harbor, pp 145–151 (Cancer Cells Series, vol 3)
6. Arimura A, Fishback JB (1981) Somatostatin: regulation of secretion. Neuroendocrinology 33:246–256
7. Arnold R, Lankisch PG (1980) Somatostatin and the gastrointestinal tract. Clin Gastroenterol 9:733–753
8. Barnes AJ, Long RG, Adrian TE, Vale W, Brown MR, Rivier JE, Hanley J, Ghatei MA, Sarson DL, Bloom SR (1981) Effect of a long-acting octapeptide analogue of somatostatin on growth hormone and pancreatic and gastrointestinal hormones in man. Clin Sci 61:653–656
9. Baxter JN, Jenkins SA, Day DW, Shields R (1985) Effect of a somatostatin analogue on hepatic and splenic RE function in the rat. Br J Surg 72:1005–1008
10. Boom SR, Poldak JM (1987) Somatostatin. BMJ 295:288–289
11. Bogden AE, Taylor JE, Moreau JP, Coy DH, Moreau S, LePage DJ (1988) In vivo responsiveness of human and animal tumours to somatostatin (SRIF) analogue BIM-23014C (DC13-116). Proc AACR 29:56
12. Bonfils S, Ruszniewski P, Costil V, Laucournet H, Vatier J, Rene E, Mignon M (1986) Prolonged treatment of Zollinger-Ellison syndrome by long-acting somatostatin. Lancet i:554
13. Brazeau P, Vale W, Burgus R (1973) Hypothalamic peptide that inhibits the secretion of immunoreactive pituitary growth hormone. Science 179:77–79
14. Charlton CDA, Parmar H, Bejot JL, Phillips RH, Lightman SL (1991) Carcinoid tumours treated with BIM 23014 (Somatuline). Eur J Can (Abstract 1918) [Suppl 2] S 312
15. Chiodini PG, Cozzi R, Dallabonanza D, Oppizzi G, Verde G, Petroncini M, Liuzzi A, Del Pozo E (1987) Medical treatment of acromegaly with SMS 201-995, a somatostatin analog: a comparison with bromocriptine. J Endocrinol Metab 64:447–453
16. Ch'ng JLC, Williams SJ, Bloom SR (1984) Chronic treatment of gut hormone producing tumours (apudomas) with a long-acting somatostatin analogue (abstract). Dig Dis Sci 29 [August suppl]:17S
17. Ch'ng JLC, Anderson JV, Williams SJ, Carr DH, Bloom SR (1986) Remission of symptoms during long-term treatment of metastatic pancreatic endocrine tumours with long acting somatostatin analog. BMJ 292:981–982
18. Christensen SE, Weeke J, Orskov H, Moller N, Flyvbjerg A, Harris AG, Lund E, Jorgensen J (1987) Continuous subcutaneous pump infusion of somatostatin analogue SMS 201-995 versus subcutaneous injection schedule in acromegalic patients. Clin Endocrinol 27:297–306
19. Clements D, Elias R (1985) Regression of metastatic VIPoma with somatostatin analog SMS 201-995. Lancet i:874–875
20. Clemmons DR, Elgin RG, Han VKM, Casella SJ, D'Ercole AJ, Van Wyk JJ (1986) Cultured fibroblast monolayers secrete a protein that alters the cellular binding of Somatomedin-C/insulin-like growth factor 1. J Clin Invest 77:1548–1556
21. Cohen MH, Creaven PJ, Fossieck BE Jr (1977) Intensive chemotherapy of small cell bronchogenic carcinoma. Cancer Treat Rep 61:349–354
22. Coy DH, Heiman ML, Rossowski J (1988) Receptor-selective somatostatin (SRIF) analogs. Proceedings of the Tenth American Peptide Symposium, p 462
23. Davis GR, Camp RC, Raskin P, Krejs GJ (1980) Effect of somatostatin infusion on jejunal water and electrolyte transport in a patient with secretory diarrhea due to malignant carcinoid syndrome. Gastroenterology 78:346–349
24. Davoren JB, Hsueh AJW (1986) Growth hormone increases ovarian levels of immunoreactive somatomedin C/insulin-like growth factor I in vivo. Endocrinology 118:888–890

25. De Quijada MG, Redding TW, Coy DH, Torres-Aleman I, Schally AV (1983) Inhibition of growth of a prolactin-secreting pituitary tumour in rats by analogs of luteinizing hormone-releasing hormone and somatostatin. Proc Natl Acad Sci USA 80:3485–3488
26. D'Ercole AJ, Stiles AD, Underwood LE (1984) Tissue concentrations of somatomedin C: further evidence for multiple sites of synthesis and paracrine or autocrine mechanisms of action. Proc Natl Acad Sci 81:935–939
27. Defeudis FV, Moreau JP (1986) Studies on somatostatin analogues might lead to new therapies for certain types of cancer. TIPS 7:384–386
28. Dembinski AB, Johnson LR (1980) Stimulation of pancreatic growth by secretin, caerulein, and pentagastrin. Endocrinology 106:323–328
29. Devrode MA, Tseng LYH, Katsoyannis PG, Nissley SP, Rechler MM (1986) Modulation of insulin-like growth factor 1 binding to human fibroblast monolayer culture by insulin-like growth factor carrier proteine released to the incubation media. J Clin Invest 77:602–613
30. Elkhammas EA, Gower WR Jr, Knierem TH, Ellison EC, Fabri PJ (1986) Biphasic response of hyperplastic G-cells to somatostatin analog (abstract). Gastroenterology 90 [Suppl 12]:1405
31. Ellison EC, Garner WI, Mekhijian HS, O'Dorisio TM, Carey LC (1986) Successful treatment of pancreatic ascites with somatostatin analog 201-995 (abstract). Gastroenterology 90 [Suppl 12]:1405
32. Ellison EC, O'Doristo TM, Elkammas E, Mekhjian HS, Sparks J (1986) Long-acting somatostatin analog inhibits calcium and secretin stimulated gastrin release in the Zollinger-Ellison syndrome (abstract). Gastroenterology 90 [Suppl 12]:1405
33. Ellison EC, O'Dorisio TM, Sparks J, Mekhjian HS, Fromkes JJ, Woltering EA, Carey LC (1986) Observations on the effect of a somatostatin analog in the Zollinger-Ellison syndrome: implications for the treatment of apudomas. Surgery 100:437–444
34. Evans WK, Osoba D, Feld R, Shepherd FA, Bazos MJ, DeBoer G (1985) Etoposide (VP-16) and cisplatin – an effective treatment for relapse in SCLC. J Clin Oncol 3:65–71
35. Fentiman IS, Brame K, Chaudary MA, Camplejohn RS, Wang DY, Millis RR (1988) Perioperative bromocriptine adjuvant treatment for operable breast cancer. Lancet i:609–610
36. Gerich JE (1981) Somatostatin and diabetes. Am J Med 70:619–626
37. Ginsberg-Fellner F, Rayfield EJ (1980) Metabolic studies in a child with a pancreatic insulinoma. Am J Dis Child 134:64–67
38. Girod C, Dubois MP, Durand N (1980) Immunocytochemical evidence for the presence of somatostatin-like immunoreactivity in scattered cells of the duct system of the submandibular glands in the monkey, Macaca irus. Histochemistry 69:137–143
39. Gomez-Pan A, Snow M, Piercy DI (1976) Actions of growth hormone-release inhibiting hormone (somatostatin) on the renin aldosterone system. J Clin Endocrinol Metab 43:240–243
40. Gonzalez-Barcena D, Rangel-Garcia NE, Perez-Sanchez PL, Gutierrez-Damperio C, Garcia-Carrasco F, Comaru-Schally AM, Schally AV (1986) Response to D-Trp-6-LHRH in advanced adenocarcinoma of pancreas (letter). Lancet ii:154
41. Goodman RH, Jacobs JW, Dee PC, Habener JF (1982) Somatostatin 28 encoded in a cloned cDNA obtained from a rat medullary thyroid carcinoma. J Biol Chem 257:1156–1159
42. Goustin AS, Leof EB, Shipley GD, Moses HL (1986) Growth factors and cancer. Cancer Res 46:1015–1029
43. Haeder M, Rotsch M, Bepler G, Henning C, Havemann K, Heimann B, Moelling K (1988) Epidermal growth factor receptor expression in human lung cancer cell lines. Cancer Res 48:1132–1136
44. Heiman ML, Murphy WA, Coy DH (1987) Differential binding of somatostatin agonists to somatostatin receptors in brain and adenohypophysis. Neuroendocrinol 45:429–436

45. Heldin CH, Westermark B (1984) Growth factors: mechanism of action and relation to oncogenes. Cell 37:9–20
46. Hierowski MT, Liebow C, Du Sapin K, Schally AV (1985) Stimulation by somatostatin of dephosphorylation of membrane proteins in pancreatic cancer MIA PaCa-2 cell line. FEBS 179:252–256
47. Hildebrandt G, Zierski J, Müller H (1987) Another approach to medical treatment of acromegaly – continuous chronic intravenous application of SMS 201-995 via implantable pump system. J Endocrinol Invest 10 [Suppl 4]:93
48. Holley RW, Böhlen P, Fava R, Baldwin JH, Kleeman G, Armour R (1980) Purification of kidney epithelial cell growth inhibitors. Proc Natl Acad Sci USA 77:5989–5992
49. Iversen OH (1985) What is new in endogenous growth stimulators and inhibitors (chalones). Path Res Pract 180:77–80
50. Johnson LR (1981) Effects of gastrointestinal hormones on pancreatic growth. Cancer 47:1640–1645
51. Kadar T, Redding TW, Ben-David M, Schally AV (1988) Receptors for prolactin, somatostatin and luteinizing hormone-releasing hormone in experimental prostate cancer after treatment with analogs of luteinizing hormone-releasing hormone and somatostatin. Proc Natl Acad Sci USA 85:890–894
52. Kirkegaard P, Olsen PS, Nexo E, Holst JJ, Poulsen SS (1984) Effect of vasoactive intestinal polypeptide and somatostatin on secretion of epidermal growth factor and bicarbonate from Brunner's glands. Gut 25:1225–1229
53. Kraenzlin ME, Ch'ng JLC, Wood SM, Carr DH, Bloom SR (1985) Long-term treatment of a VIPoma with somatostatin analogue resulting in remission of symptoms and possible shrinkage of metastases. Gastroenterology 88:185–187
54. Krisch B (1981) Somatostatin-immunoreactive fiber projections into the brain stem and the spinal cord of the rat. Cell Tissue Res 217:531–552
55. Krisch B (1987) Hypothalamic and extrahypothalamic distribution of somatostatin-immunoreactive elements in the rat brain. Cell Tissue Res 195:499–513
56. Kvols LK, Moertel CG, O'Connell MJ, Schutt AJ, Rubin J, Hahn RG (1986) Treatment of the malignant carcinoid syndrome: evaluation of a long-acting somatostatin analogue. N Engl J Med 345:663–666
57. Lamberts SWJ, Uitterlinden P, Zuiderwijk J, Verleun T, Neufeld M, Del Pozo E (1984) The effects of a long-acting somatostatin analog on pituitary tumour growth and hormone secretion in rat and man. 7th International Congress of Endocrinology, Quebec City. Excerpta Medica, Amsterdam
58. Lamberts SW, Oosterom R, Neufeld M, Del Pozo E (1985) The somatostatin analog SMS 201-995 induces long-acting inhibition of growth hormone secretion without rebound hypersecretion in acromegalic patients. J Clin Endocrinol Metab 60(6):1161–1165
59. Lamberts SW, Uitterlinden P, Verschoor L, Van Dougen KJ, Del Pozo E (1985) Long-term treatment of acromegaly with the somatostatin analogue SMS 201-995. N Eng J Med 313(25):1575–1580
60. Lamberts SWJ, Zweens M, Verschoor L, Del Pozo E (1986) A comparison among the growth hormone-lowering effects in acromegaly of the somatostatin analog SMS 201-995, bromocriptine, and the combination of both drugs. J Clin Endocrinol Metab 63:16–19
61. Lamberts SWJ, Koper JW, Reubi JC (1987) Potential role of somatostatin analogues in the treatment of cancer. Eur J Clin Invest 17:281–287
62. Lewin MJ (1986) Somatostatin receptors. Scand J Gastroenterol [Suppl] 119:42–46
63. Liebow C, Hierowski M, DuSapin K (1986) Hormonal control of pancreatic cancer growth. Pancreas 1:44–48
64. Lippman ME, Dickson RB, Kasid A, Gelmann E, Davidson N; McManaway M, Huff K, Bronzert D, Bates S, Swain S, Knabbe C (1986) Autocrine and paracrine growth regulation of human breast cancer. J Steroid Biochem 24:147–154
65. Long RG, Barnes AJ, Adrian TE, Mallinson CN, Brown MR, Vale W, Rivier JE, Christofides ND, Bloom SR (1979) Suppression of pancreatic endocrine tumour secretion by long-acting somatostatin analogue. Lancet ii:764–767

66. Longnecker SM (1988) Somatostatin and octreotide: literature review and description of therapeutic activity in pancreatic neoplasia. Drug Intell Clin Pharm 22:99–105
67. Macauly VM, Teale JD, Everard MJ, Joshi GP, Smith IE, Millar JL (1987) Somatostatin-C/insulin-like growth factor-I is a mitogen for human small cell lung cancer. Br J Cancer 57:91–93
68. Mandarino L, Stenner D, Blanchard W (1981) Selective effects of somatostatin-14, -25 and -28 on in vitro insulin and glucagon secretion. Nature 291:76–77
69. Marbach P, Neufeld M, Pless J (1985) Clinical Applications of Somatostatin Analogues. Adv Exp Med Biol 188:339–353
70. Mascardo RN, Sherline P (1982) Somatostatin inhibits rapid centrosomal separation and cell proliferation induced by epidermal growth factor. Endocrinology 3:1394–1396
71. Maton PN, O'Dorisio TM, Howe BA, McArthur KE, Howard JM, Cherner JA, Malarkey TB, Collen MJ, Gardner JD, Jensen RT (1985) Effect of a long-acting somatostatin analogues (SMS 201-995) in a patient with pancreatic cholera. N Engl J Med 312:17–21
72. Matuo Y, Nishi N, Matsui S, Sandberg AA, Isaacs JT, Wada F (1987) Heparin binding affinity of rat prostatic growth factor in normal and cancerous prostates: Partial purification and characterization of rat prostatic growth factor in the Dunning tumour. Cancer Res 47(1):188–192
73. McCann SM, Krulich L, Negro-Vilar A, Ojeda SR, Vijayan E (1980) Regulation and function of panhibin (somatostatin). Adv Biochem Psychopharmacol 22:131–143
74. McCumbee WD, Lebovitz H (1980) Hormone responsiveness of a transplantable rat chondrosarcoma. In vitro effects of growth hormone dependent serum factors and insulin. Endocrinology 106:905–910
75. McGuire WL, Dressler LG, Owens M, Seamer L (1986) Identifying breast cancer patients for adjuvant therapy by DNA flow cytometry and steroid receptors: A 1000 patient study. 14th International Cancer Congress Proceedings I, p 20
76. McKeehan WL, Adams PS, Fast D (1987) Different hormonal requirements for androgen-independent growth of normal and tumour epithelial cells from rat prostate. In Vitro Cell Dev Biol 23(2):147–152
77. Mee AD, Khan O, Mashiter K (1984) High serum prolactin associated with poor prognosis in carcinoma of the prostate. Br J Urol 56:698–701
78. Miller RE (1981) Pancreatic neuroendocrinology: peripheral neural mechanism in the regulation of the islets of Langerhans. Endocr Rev 2:471–494
79. Moreau JP, DeFeudis FV (1987) Pharmacological studies of somatostatin and somatostatin-analogues: therapeutic advances and perspectives. Life Sci 40:419–437
80. Murphy WA, Lance VA, Moreau S, Moreau JP, Coy DH (1987) Inhibition of rat prostate tumour growth by an octapeptide analog of somatostatin. Life Sci 40:2515–2522
81. Nilsson A, Isgaard J, Lindahl A, Dahlström A, Skottner A, Isaksson OGP (1986) Regulation by growth hormone of number of chondrocytes containing IGF-I in rat growth plate. Science 233:571–574
82. Nott DM, Baxter JN, Day DW, Cooke TG, Jenkins SA (1987) The effect of SMS 201-995 on the growth and development of hepatic metastases. Br J Surg 74:1162
83. Parmar H, Phillips RH, Lightman SL, Edwards L, Allen L, Schally AV (1985) Randomised controlled study of orchidectomy vs long acting D-Trp-6-LHRH microcapsules in advanced prostatic carcinoma. Lancet ii:1201–1205
84. Parmer H, Nicoll J, Stockdale A, Cassoni A, Phillips RH, Lightman SL, Schally AV (1985) Advanced ovarian carcinoma: response to the agonist D-Trp-6-LHRH. Cancer Treat Rep 69:1341–1342
85. Parmar H, Edwards L, Phillips RH, Allen L, Lightman SL (1987) Orchiectomy vs long-acting D-Trp-6-LHRH in advanced prostatic cancer. Br J Urol 59(3):248–254
86. Parmar H, Phillips RH, Rustin G, Lightman SL, Schally AV (1988) Therapy of advanced ovarian cancer with D-Trp-6-LHRH (Decapeptyl) microcapsules. Biomed Pharmacother 42:531–538

87. Parmar H, Rustin G, Lightman SL, Phillips RH, Hanham IW, Schally AV (1988) Response to D-Trp-6-LHRH (Decapeptyl) microcapsules in advanced ovarian cancer. BMJ 296:1229
88. Parmar H, Bogden A, Mollard M, De Rouge B, Phillips RH, Lightman SL (1989) Somatostatin and somatostatin analogues in oncology. Cancer Treat Rev 16:95–115
89. Parmar H, Charlton C, Bejot JL, Phillips RH, Edwards L, Lightman SL (1991) BIM 23014 (Somatuline) in advanced prostate cancer. Eur J Cancer [Suppl 2] S116 (Abstract)
90. Parmar H, Charlton CDA, Phillips RH, Edwards L, Bejot JL, Thomas F, Lightman SL (1992) Therapeutic response to somatostatin analogue, BIM 23014 in metastatic prostate cancer. Clin Exp Metastasis 10:3–11
91. Pawlkowski M, Zelazowski P, Stepien H, Schally AV (1987) Somatostatin and its analog enhance the formation of human leukocyte migration inhibiting factor: further evidence for immunomodulatory action of somatostatin. Peptides 8:951–952
92. Paz-Bouza JI, Redding TW, Schally AV (1987) Treatment of nitrosamine-induced pancreatic tumours in hamsters with analogs of somatostatin and luteinizing hormone-releasing hormone. Proc Natl Acad Sci USA 84:1112–1116
93. Peehl DM, Stamey TA (1986) Growth responses of normal, benign hyperplastic and malignant human prostatic epithelial cells in vitro to cholera toxin, pituitary extract and hydrocortisone. Prostate 8(1):51–61
94. Peehl DM, Stamey TA (1986) Serum-free growth of adult human prostatic epithelial cells. In Vitro Cell Dev Biol 22(2):82–90
95. Pelletier G (1980) Immunohistochemical localization of somatostatin. Prog Histochem Cytochem 12(3):1–41
96. Perry MC, Eaton WL, Propert KJ, Ware JH, Zimmer B, Chahinian AP, Skarin A, Carey RW, Kreisman H, Faulkner C (1987) Chemotherapy with or without radiation therapy in limited small cell carcinoma of the lung. N Engl J Med 316:912–918
97. Petersen H, Solomon T, Grossman MI (1978) Effect of chronic pentagastrin, cholecystokinin, and secretin on pancreas of rats. American Physiological Society, pp E286–E293
98. Polak J, Pearse AGE, Grimelins L, Bloom S, Arimura A (1975) Growth-hormone release-inhibiting hormone in gastrointestinal and pancreatic D cells. Lancet i:1220–1222
99. Redding TW, Schally AV (1982) Inhibition of cell growth by a hypothalamic peptide. Proc Natl Acad Sci USA 79:7014–7018
100. Redding TW, Schally AV (1983) Inhibition of growth of the transplantable rat chondrosarcoma by analogs of hypothalamic hormones. Proc Natl Acad Sci USA 80:1078–1082
101. Redding TW, Schally AV (1984) Inhibition of growth of pancreatic carcinomas in animal models by analogs of hypothalamic hormones. Proc Natl Acad Sci USA 81:248–252
102. Reichlin S (1981) Systems for the study of regulation of neuropeptide secretion. Adv Biochem Psychopharmacol 28:573–597
103. Reichlin S (1983) Somatostatin. N Engl J Med 309(24):1495–1501
104. Reichlin S (1983) Somatostatin. N Engl J Med 309(25):1556–1563
105. Reid IA, Rose JC (1977) An intrarenal effect of somatostatin on water excretion. Endocrinology 100:782–785
106. Rene E, Bonfils S (1984) Control of severe diarrhea with somatostatin (letter). N Engl J Med 311:598
107. Reubi JC (1985) A somatostatin analogue inhibits chondrosarcoma and insulinoma tumour growth. Acta Endocrinologica 109:108–114
108. Reubi JC, Maurer R, Klijn JGM, Stefando SZ, Foekens JA, Blaauw G, Blankenstein MA, Lamberts SWJ (1986) High incidence of somatostatin receptors in human meningiomas: biochemical characterization. J Clin Endocrinol Metab 63:433–437
109. Reubi JC, Maurer R, Von Werder K, Torhorst J, Klijn JGM, Lamberts SWJ (1987) Somatostatin receptors in human endocrine tumours. Cancer Res 47:551–558
110. Rose DP, Gottardis M, Noonan JJ (1983) Rat mammary carcinoma regressions during suppression of serum growth hormone and prolactin. Anticancer Res 3:323–326

111. Sainsbury JRC, Farndon JR, Needham GK, Malcolm AJ, Harris AL (1987) Epidermal-growth-factor receptor status as predictor of early recurrence of and death from breast cancer. Lancet i:1398–1402
112. Scambia G, Panici PB, Baiocchi G, Perrone L, Iacobelli S (1988) Antiproliferative effects of somatostatin and the somatostatin analog SMS 201-995 on three human breast cancer cell lines. J Cancer Res Clin Oncol 114:306–308
113. Schally AV, Redding TW (1987) Somatostatin analogs as adjuncts to agonists of luteinizing hormone-releasing hormone in the treatment of experimental prostate cancer. Proc Natl Acad Sci USA 84:7275–7279
114. Setyono-Han B, Henkelman MS, Foekens JA, Klijn JGM (1987) Direct inhibitory effects of somatostatin (analogues) on the growth of human breast cancer cells. Cancer Res 47:1566–1570
115. Shepherd JJ, Senator GB (1986) Regression of liver metastases in patient with gastrin-secreting tumour treated with SMS 201-995. Lancet ii:574
116. Sherwin SA, Minna JD, Gazdar F, Todaro GJ (1981) Expression of epidermal and nerve growth factor receptors and soft agar growth factor production by human lung cancer cells. Cancer Res 41:3538–3542
117. Smith JJ, Derynck R, Korc M (19897) Production of transforming growth factor alpha in human pancreatic cancer cells: evidence for a superagonist autocrine cycle. Proc Natl Acad Sci USA 84:7567–7570
118. Smith RG, Syms AJ, Nag A, Lerner S, Norris JS (1985) Mechanism of the glucocorticoid regulation of growth of the androgen-sensitive prostate-derived R3327H-G8-Al tumour cell line. J Biol Chem 260(23):12454–12463
119. Sporn MB, Roberts AB (1986) Peptide growth factors and inflammation, tissue repair, and cancer. J Clin Invest 78:329
120. Sporn MB, Todaro GJ (1980) Autocrine secretion and malignant transformation of cells. N Engl J Med 303:378–389
121. Stöckmann F, Richter G, Conlon JM, Lembcke B, Creutzfeldt W (1986) Effect of short- and long-term treatment with SMS 201-995 in patients with carcinoid tumours. Gastroenterology 90 [Suppl 2] 1650
122. Stoscheck CM, King LE Jr (1986) Role of epidermal growth factor in carcinogenesis. Cancer Res 46:1030–1037
123. Taylor JE, Bogden AE, Moreau JP, Coy DH (1988) In vitro and in vivo inhibition of human small cell lung carcinoma (NCI-H69) growth by a somatostatin analogue. Biochem Biophys Res Comm 153:81–86
124. Taylor JE, Coy DH, Moreau JP (1988) High affinity binding of 125-Tyr11 somatostatin 14 to human small cell carcinoma (NC1-H69). Biochem Biophys Res Comm (in press)
125. Theve ON, Pousette A, Carlstrom K (1983) Adenocarcinoma of the pancreas – a hormone sensitive tumour? A preliminary report on noraldex treatment. Clin Oncol 9:193–197
126. Todaro GJ, Fryling C, De Larco JE (1980) Transforming growth factors produced by certain human tumour cells: polypeptides that interact with epidermal growth factor receptors. Proc Natl Acad Sci USA 77:5258–5262
127. Tolis G, Yotis A, Del Pozo E, Pitoulis S (1986) Therapeutic efficacy of a somatostatin analogues (SMS 201-995) in active acromegaly. J Neurosurg 65:37–40
128. Venier A, De Simone C, Forni L, Ghirlanda G, Uccioli L, Serri F, Frati L (1988) Treatment of severe psoriasis with somatostatin: four years of experience. Arch Dermatol Res 280 [Suppl]:S51–S54
129. Von Werder K, Losa M, Müller AO, Schweiberer L, Fahlbusch R, Del Pozo E (1984) Treatment of metastasing GRF-producing tumour with a long-acting somatostatin analogue. Lancet ii:282–283
130. Wagner H, Hengst K, Zierden E, Gerlach U (1978) Investigations of the antiproliferative effect of somatostatin in man and rats. Metabolism 27 [Suppl 1]:1381
131. Wahl MI, Carpenter G (1987) Role of growth factors and their receptors in the control of normal cell proliferation and cancer. Clin Physiol Biochem 5:130–139

132. Weber MM, Chaproniere-Rickenberg DM, Donhbue RE (1983) Insulin, EGF and glucocorticoids in the regulation of growth in normal and neoplastic human prostatic epithelial cells (Meeting abstract). Proc Am Assoc Cancer Res 24:719
133. Williams G, Burrin JM, Ball JA, Joplin GF, Bloom SR (1986) Effective and lasting growth hormone suppression in active acromegaly with oral administration of somatostatin analog SMS 201-995. Lancct ii:774–778
134. Williams NS, Cooper JC, Axon ATR, King RFG, Barker M (1984) Use of a long acting somatostatin analogue in controlling life threatening ileostomy diarrhoea. Br Med J 289:1027–1028
135. Woll PJ, Rozengurt E (1988) Bombesin and bombesin antagonists: Studies in Swiss 3T3 cells and human small cell lung cancer. Br J Cancer 57:579–586
136. Wood SM, Polak JM, Bloom SR (1983) Gut hormone secreting tumours. Scand J Gastroenterol [Suppl] 82:165–179
137. Wood SM, Kraenzlin ME, Adrian TE, Bloom SR (1985) Treatment of patients with pancreatic endocrine tumours using a new long-acting somatostatin analogue symptomatic and peptide responses. Gut 26:438–444
138. Zezulak KM, Green H (1986) The generation of insulin-like growth factor-I-sensitive cells by growth hormone action. Science 233:551–553
139. Zimmerman PV, Hawson T, Bint MH, Parsons PG (1987) Ploidy as a prognostic determinant in surgically treated lung cancer. Lancet ii:530–533
140. Zuiderwijk J, Verleun T, Neufeld M, Del Pozo E (1984) The effects of a long-acting somatostatin analog on pituitary tumour growth and hormone secretion in rat and man. 7th International Congress of Endocrinology (Quebec). Excerpta Medica Amsterdam, p 847

Somatostatin Analogues in Pituitary Adenomas

K. von Werder

Schloßparkklinik, Freie Universität Berlin, Heubnerweg 2, 1000 Berlin 19, FRG

Introduction

Evidence that the secretion of growth hormone (GH) is under the dual control of a hypothalamic stimulating hormone – growth hormone releasing hormone (GHRH) – and an inhibitory factor was already presented by Krulich et al. in 1968. However, only in 1973 did Brazeau et al. isolate a tetradecapeptide from ovine hypothalami that inhibited GH or somatotropin secretion. The peptide was called somatostatin or growth-hormone release-inhibiting hormone.

Subsequent work revealed that somatostatin is not only present in the hypothalamus or the central nervous system, but also in many tissues outside the brain, particularly the intestinal tract (Reichlin 1983). Since somatostatin plays a physiologic role as both a hypophysiotropic and a gastrointestinal inhibitory hormone, it was considered to be potentially useful as a therapeutic agent soon after its discovery (Chiodini et al. 1991). However, its therapeutic use was precluded by the rapid enzymatic breakdown which was responsible for its very short half-life in blood (Reichlin 1983).

After reports were published that an octapeptide analog of somatostatin had full biological activity (Sassolas and Melmed 1992), a rational drug design was started in order to develop a compound with a longer biological half-life and possibly a more specific inhibitory effect on the pituitary than on the endocrine pancreas. In 1982, Bauer and co-workers in the Sandoz Research Laboratories had synthesized an octapeptide which was extraordinarily resistant to metabolic degradation. This peptide, with the clinical code SMS 201-995, was later called octreotide and was found to be particularly suitable for therapeutic use in patients with acromegaly and gastroenteropancreatic tumors. In the meantime, the therapeutic use of this analog has extended to include a wide range of diseases. Thus, the potential for octreotide treatment has escalated in the past few years, although adequate clinical studies are often still required before the indication for octreotide for a particular endocrine disease can be established (von Werder and Faglia 1992); this does not, however, pertain to GH-secreting tumours which now represent a well-established

Recent Results in Cancer Research, Vol. 129

indication for octreotide treatment (Barkan et al. 1988; Ching et al. 1985; Chiodini et al. 1987; Lamberts et al. 1985, 1986, 1987; Quabbe and Plöckinger 1989; Sassolas 1992). In addition, octreotide therapy has become established in the rare thyroid stimulating hormone (TSH)-producing pituitary adenomas (Chanson and Warnet 1992). In contrast to GH- and TSH-producing tumors, other pituitary tumors such as prolactin (PRL)-, adrenocorticotrophic (ACTH)- and gonadotropin-producing adenomas or nonfunctioning tumors of the pituitary rarely respond to octreotide treatment (von Werder and Faglia 1992).

In the following, octreotide treatment of GH-secreting tumors will be discussed first, followed by a review of the literature on octreotide treatment of TSH-producing tumors. Finally, the efficacy of octreotide in the treatment of endocrine-inactive pituitary tumours, in patients with Cushing's syndrome and in those with prolactinomas will be discussed.

Octreotide Treatment of Acromegaly

Clinical interest in an effective medical treatment of GH-secreting tumors is based on the experience that the elevated GH levels found in patients with acromegaly are frequently not normalized by surgery or radiotherapy (Harris 1991; von Werder 1985; von Werder et al. 1987). Bromocriptine and later other dopamine (DA) agonists which have been shown to lower GH levels (Liuzzi et al. 1974) have been used in those patients who did not respond to surgery or still had elevated GH levels after radiotherapy. However, DA agonists have certain drawbacks: they reduce GH levels in only about half of patients, and normalization of GH levels occurs in less than 20% of them (von Werder et al. 1987). In addition, adenoma shrinkage, which is observed in 85% of all patients with prolactinomas during DA agonist therapy (Bevan et al. 1992), is rarely found in patients with acromegaly, who often have large tumors. Lastly, even after prolonged treatment with DA agonists, withdrawal of the drug is followed by a rapid reincrease of GH levels to the former basal values (Besser and Wass 1987; Bevan et al. 1992).

For this reason, medical treatment with dopaminergic compounds is generally considered as an additive approach when other more radical forms of treatment have failed (von Werder et al. 1987). When octreotide became available for clinical investigation, it was soon demonstrated that it could effectively reduce elevated GH levels in patients with acromegaly (Lamberts et al. 1985). This was not surprising since soon after the discovery of native somatostatin it could be shown that constant intravenous infusion of the tetradecapeptide led to prompt inhibition of GH levels, followed by a rebound immediately after the infusion was stopped (von Werder 1975). Furthermore, using an autoradiographic technique, Reubi et al. (1987) demonstrated receptors for labeled octreotide at the somatotroph adenomatous cells of GH-secreting tumors. In fact it could be demonstrated that the GH-lowering effect of octreotide in acromegaly patients in vivo correlated with the somatostatin receptor status of the adenoma in vitro (Reubi and Landolt 1989). More recently, using indium-labeled octreotide (Octreoscan, Mallinckrodt, Petten, Holland), these receptors could be visualized in vivo (Lamberts et al. 1990).

Effect on GH and IGF-I Levels

The octapeptide analog of naturally occurring somatostatin proved to be 45 times more active in inhibiting GH activity, but only 1.3 times more active in inhibiting insulin secretion than native somatostatin (Sassolas and Melmed 1992). This makes the compound particularly useful for treating hypersecretion of GH. Acute injection of 50–100 µg octreotide (Sandostatin) in acromegaly patients leads in most cases to a rapid fall in GH levels, with the nadir occurring 3 h after injection (Lamberts et al. 1985; Mehltretter et al. 1991). GH levels remain significantly suppressed for 10 h, after which there is a steady rise to the preinjection level within 2 h, but without the rebound phenomena that are observed with the native peptide (Reichlin 1983).

The acute effect persists during chronic administration of octreotide. Studies of daily GH profiles show that subcutaneous administration of 100 µg octreotide three times per day prevents the increase of GH levels to above 5 ng/ml (Lamberts et al. 1985; Mehltretter et al. 1991) (Fig. 1). An increase to

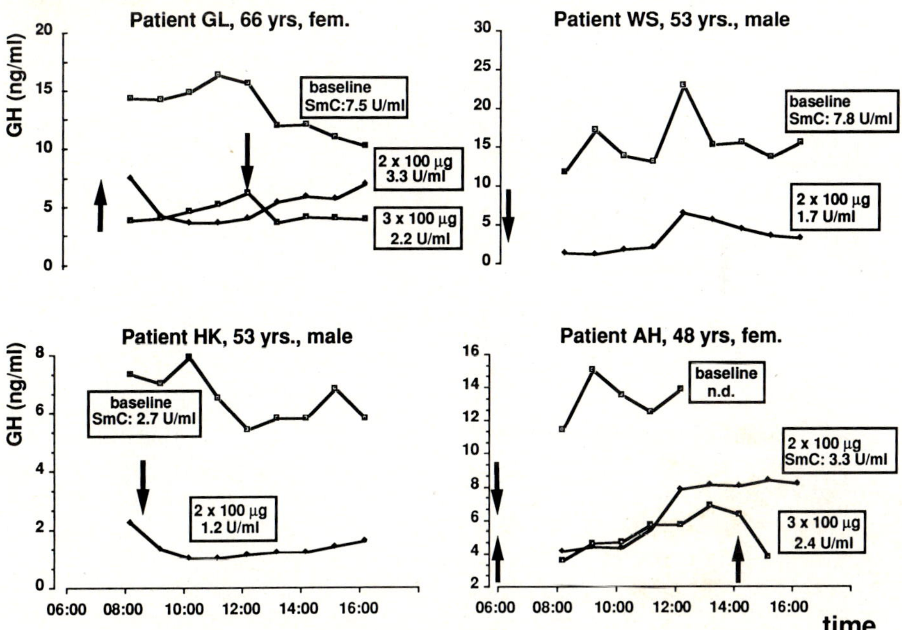

Fig. 1. Growth hormone (*GH*) levels of patients responding to octreotide treatment. The *arrows* (↑↓) indicate time of injection of 100 µg octreotide for each patient. In the *boxes* the daily dose regimen and corresponding IGF-I levels are shown. (From Mehltretter et al. 1991)

above this level would occur in a number of patients if the daily dose were administered in only two injections (Mehltretter et al. 1991). Although even with three daily injections GH fluctuations exceeding the normal range can be observed, insulin-like growth factor I (IGF-I) levels are often normalized (Lamberts et al. 1987; Sassolas et al. 1990).

Current experience of octreotide treatment in acromegalic patients extends to more than 500 cases. The largest series has been compiled by Vance and Harris (1991), who have collected together information on 189 acromegaly patients from many centers all over the world. Most therapeutic trials have been performed with 100 µg octreotide administered three times daily, a dosage which seems optimal for the majority of acromegaly patients. However, higher dosages of up to 500 µg three times daily have occasionally been required to effectively lower GH levels in some acromegaly patients (Quabbe and Plöckinger 1989; Mehltretter et al. 1991). Even these dosages do not lead to normalization of GH levels or GH-dependent IGF-I production in all acromegaly patients (Fig. 2). Indeed, some patients, albeit a small minority, do not show any change in GH levels during octreotide treatment (Mehltretter et al. 1991) (Table 1).

Considerable variability in the sensitivity of GH secretion to somatostatin has been demonstrated in vitro and in vivo for acromegaly patients. Using a reverse hemolytic plaque assay, Hofland et al. (1989) demonstrated a marked heterogeneity of pituitary adenoma cell subpopulations with corresponding GH release in patients with acromegaly. According to Hofland et al. (1989), adenoma cells that form large GH plaques are particularly sensitive to octreotide. Furthermore, the therapeutic effectivity of octreotide in acromegaly patients correlated with the adenoma's somatostatin receptor status (Reubi

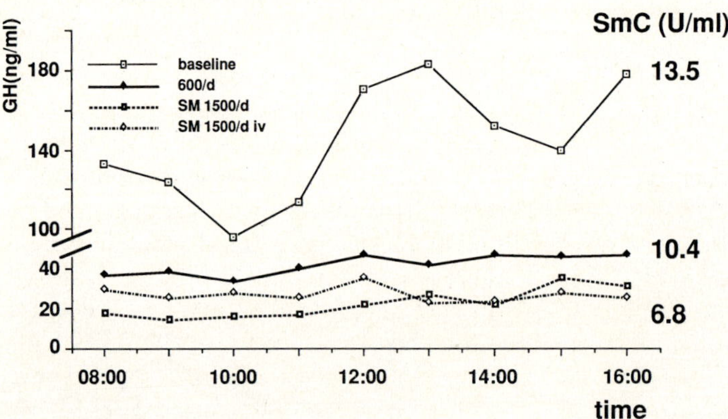

Fig. 2. Effect of octreotide (*SM*) in a 29-year-old female patient with acromegaly. The patient had been operated on three times, irradiated, and received 30 mg bromocriptine per day. Even high dosages of octreotide did not lead to normalization of GH and IGF-I (*SmC*) levels, although a significant reduction of both parameters could be observed. There was no difference between subcutaneous and intravenous administration of 1500 µg octreotide over 24 h

Table 1. Median and range of mean GH and IGF-I levels before and during optimum therapy with octreotide

Group	Before octreotide		During octreotide		Reduction of baseline (%)	
	GH (μg/L)	IGF-I (U/ml)	GH (μg/L)	IGF-I (U/ml)	GH	IGF-I
A ($n = 4$)	13.1; 6.4–15.2	7.5; 3.8–7.8	4.4; 1.2–4.6	2.0; 1.1–2.4	66.4	73.3
B ($n = 10$)	22.1; 11.8–146.7	8.5; 3.7–13.5	4.8; 2.9–23.0	2.7; 1.6–5.6	78.3	68.2
C ($n = 3$)	10.3; 9.4–11.6	9.4; 5.8–10.0	9.3; 7.7–10.6	5.0; 4.8–7.1	9.7	46.2

and Landolt 1989): the best in vivo responses occurred in patients whose tumors contained a high density of homogeneously distributed receptors with high octreotide affinity. Whether patients who do not respond adequately to octreotide may also have reduced sensitivity due to disturbed somatostatin receptor function is not clear.

In the international, multicenter, acromegaly treatment study with octreotide reported by Harris et al. (1988), it was shown that most of the 178 acromegaly patients treated with different doses of octreotide (100–1500 μg/day) and for different lengths of time experienced a significant reduction in GH levels: these fell by more than 50% in 87% of patients, to below 10 ng/ml in 75% of patients, and to below 5 ng/ml in 46% of patients. No rebound GH hypersecretion was observed after therapy ceased. Furthermore, there was no evidence of any escape from GH suppression during an observation time of up to 34 months (Harris et al. 1988). IGF-I levels were normalized in 36% of the 165 patients studied.

These observations concur with the results of other individual or multicenter trials that have since been reported (summarized in Harris 1991). However, there are obviously selected patients in whom the effect of octreotide on GH levels is less pronounced. Mehltretter et al. (1991) reported normalization of GH and IGF-I levels in only four out of 17 patients who were otherwise resistant to other forms of treatment (surgery, radiotherapy, or bromocriptine). In ten patients, there was a fall in GH and IGF-I levels, although not to within the normal range, despite the fact that higher dosages of up to 1500 μg/day were used (Fig. 2). In three of these 17 patients, octreotide had no effect on GH levels, even when the dosage was raised to 1500 μg per day and administered as a continuous subcutaneous infusion (Table 1). The latter method of administration was shown to be more effective in some patients than the conventional treatment in which the daily dosage was divided into three subcutaneous injections (Christensen et al. 1987; James et al. 1989; Mehltretter et al. 1991).

Since the response of GH levels to acute administration of octreotide in patients with acromegaly is predictive of the response to long-term therapy (Lamberts et al. 1988), patients who fail to respond to the acute injection of 50 μg octreotide should not be treated with the compound (Lamberts et al.

1985, Mehltretter et al. 1991). In fact, there is a close correlation between the mean GH level reached 2–6 h after a single subcutaneous injection of 50 µg octreotide and the minimal level achieved during chronic therapy (Fig. 3). In addition, a good correlation between the mean 24-h GH levels and IGF-I levels was demonstrated, which indicates that IGF-I is a very sensitive indicator for GH hypersecretion and the success of therapy. This pertains also to other forms of treatment, e.g., after transsphenoidal surgery normal IGF-I levels were only found in patients who had adequate glucose suppressibility of GH levels to less than 2 ng/ml (Losa et al. 1989). However, in addition to lowering IGF-I levels, octreotide also stimulates IGF-binding protein 1 (IGF-BP-1), which competes with the IGF-I receptor and attenuates IGF-I action (Ezzat et al. 1992).

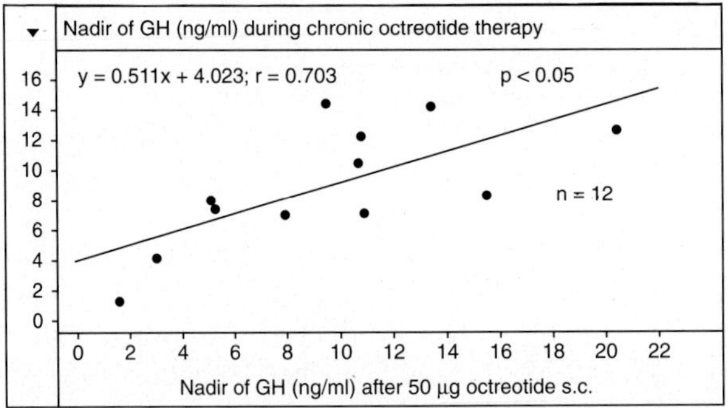

Fig. 3. Correlation between maximal suppression of growth hormone (*GH*) levels after a single dosage of octreotide and during long-term therapy

The completeness of suppression of GH secretion during octreotide treatment can also be demonstrated by the suppression of GH responses to GHRH and thyrotropin-releasing hormone (TRH) (Pieters et al. 1987). Recently, other somatostatin analogs have been developed which can be bound to microspheres (Heron et al. 1992). After intramuscular injection, a long-lasting inhibition of GH levels for up to 14 days can be achieved (Heron et al. 1992). Large doses of somatostatin analogus can be administered by this route, leading to further lowering of GH levels in patients with a subnormal response to conventional octreotide treatment (Schopohl et al. 1993). A further advantage is the fact that, instead of three subcutaneous injections per day, the analog can be administered intramuscularly only once a week (Schopohl et al. 1993).

Effect on Clinical Features

Specific symptoms of acromegaly such as headaches, sweating, soft tissue swelling, paresthesias, and arthralgias were found to be relieved within the first days of treatment (Harris 1991). Significant and rapid clinical improvement was seen in up to 87% of patients, regardless of the dosage of octreotide used. Particularly headache, which is a common and severe symptom in acromegaly, often disappears within a few minutes, suggesting that octreotide has a specific analgesic effect, independent of GH suppression (Chrubasik et al. 1984).

About 50% of acromegaly patients suffer from arthropathy. With a significant reduction of soft tissue swelling, moderate improvement of arthropathy has been observed (Harris 1991). Furthermore, sleep apnea can be improved, and beneficial effects on cardiac function can be noted in acromegaly patients after octreotide therapy. For example, a few weeks of treatment with octreotide has been observed to lead to recovery of normal physical activity, the previously used therapy for heart failure could be reduced, and the heart size normalized, as documented by X-ray (Harris 1991). During long-term treatment with octreotide leading to effective GH reduction, a diminution of the increased left ventricular mass can be expected.

Effect on Tumor Size

A reduction of pituitary tumor size is an important goal in the treatment of patients with acromegaly and larger tumors extending above the sella turcica. In ten patients with previously untreated acromegaly due to pituitary tumors who were treated with 150–1000 μg octreotide daily for up to 30 weeks, tumor size was reduced by 22%–54% (Stevenaert et al. 1992) (Fig. 4). In contrast to DA agonists, which are claimed to induce proliferation of fibrous tissue in lactotroph adenomas, after treatment with octreotide the adenomas were found to be more liquid and could be sucked off more easily (D. Lüdecke, personal communication).

Presurgical Therapy

The treatment of choice in acromegaly is still transsphenoidal surgery (Quabbe 1982; Ross and Wilson 1988; von Werder et al. 1987). The operative results are inversely correlated to the size of the tumor and the GH level (von Werder 1975). When octreotide leads to shrinkage of the GH-secreting adenoma, this should thus result in an improvement of the results of transsphenoidal surgery. However, in the series presented by Stevenaert et al. (1992), no effect on surgical outcome was seen, except in patients harboring enclosed adenomas, who tended to have a higher success rate (Stevenaert et al. 1992). The fact that in addition to effecting tumor shrinkage octreotide improves the clinical condition before surgery suggests that presurgical treatment with the peptide is generally beneficial to acromegaly patients. However, larger series have to be investigated in order to determine the usefulness of preoperative octreotide administration as a routine treatment.

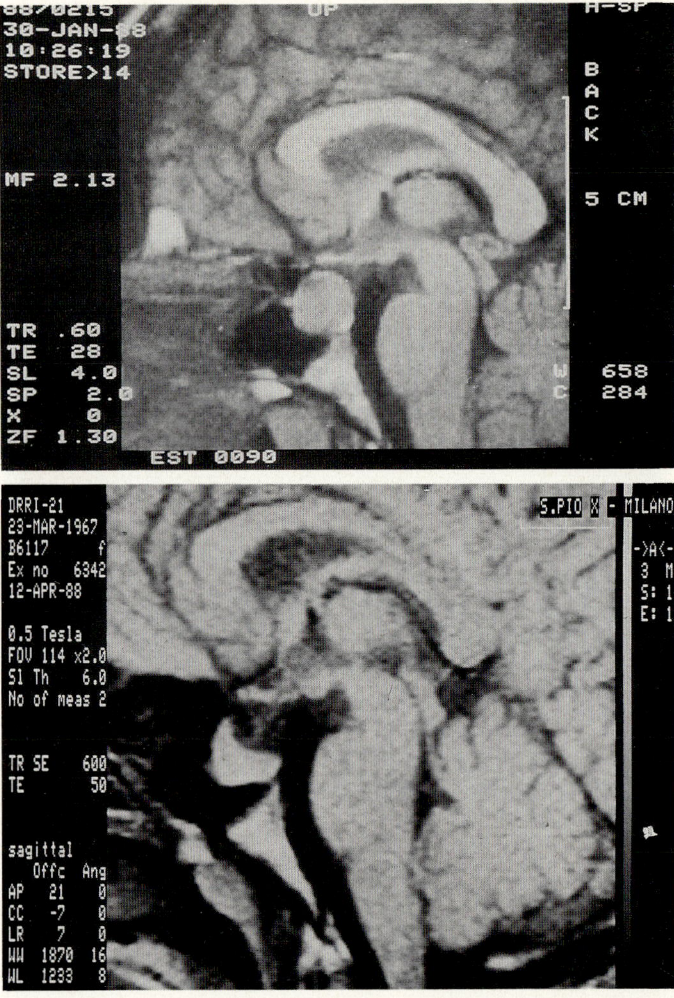

Fig. 4. Shrinkage of a GH-producing pituitary tumor (*above*) after octreotide treatment (*below*). (Courtesy of Dr. P. G. Chiodini, Milan)

Side Effects

Long-term studies demonstrate that octreotide is generally well-tolerated. However, severe diarrhea has led to discontinuation of therapy in about 2% of patients (Vance and Harris 1991; Sassolas et al. 1990). Symptoms of slight abdominal discomfort, rarely cramps, slight diarrhea and flatulence are usually encountered only at the beginning of therapy and disappear after the first week or month. However, Plöckinger et al. (1990) reported moderate to severe gastritis during chronic treatment in 9 patients who had a gastric biopsy. This indicates that patients should be closely monitored for changes in the gastric mucosa.

Glucose tolerance has been carefully studied. Somatostatin suppresses both insulin and GH secretion, effects on the carbohydrate metabolism which neutralize each other. Acute deterioration of glucose tolerance in patients with acromegaly during octreotide treatment rarely occurs (Sassolas 1992). In acromegaly patients with insulin-dependent diabetes mellitus, no change in glucose levels on hemoglobin A_{1c} levels could be observed, although often a reduction in insulin requirements was noted. In acromegaly patients with diabetes mellitus type II, worsening, improvement, or no change in glucose levels has been reported (Sassolas 1992). It is generally recommended that glucose tolerance be monitored closely, particularly at the beginning of octreotide treatment. No change in thyroid hormone or TSH levels has been reported, however, a significant reduction in the response of TSH to TRH has been observed.

Pain at the injection site has been reported in about 10% of patients. This can be minimized by slow injection and by warming up the ampules to room temperature. Development of gallstones during octreotide treatment in acromegaly is the greatest concern. There are more than ten reports in the literature dealing with this side effect, and the frequency of new gallstones developing during long-term octreotide treatment, as monitored by ultrasonography, is up to 50%. The reported prevalence of gallstones in patients treated with octreotide varies, and little is known about their incidence, composition, and pathogenetic mechanism (Dowling et al. 1992). Cholelithiasis occurring during octreotide treatment most often consists of multiple small calculi and only occasionally large gallstones. Generally, gallstone formation is associated with high doses of the drug, and the number of patients acquiring gallstones increases with duration of therapy. Most of the patients reported in the literature have no symptoms related to the presence of gallstones. However, in six patients with symptomatic cholelithiasis, cholecystectomy had to be performed, and in two patients octreotide therapy had to be stopped because of acute pancreatitis (Dowling et al. 1992).

Some patients have received ursodeoxycholic acid combined with octreotide, which led to rapid dissolution of gallstones (Buscail et al. 1989). Whether this combination treatment can be recommended is still an open question, since inhibition of gallbladder motility, impaired postprandial emptying, and changes in bile composition (oversaturation) are considered to be the major factors in the lithogenesis caused by somatostatin analogs (Dowling et al. 1992).

Octreotide and DA Agonists

Comparison of octreotide and bromocriptine was recently made in an 8-week randomized study with increasing dosages of both drugs (Halse et al. 1990). Although both groups experienced a rapid clinical response and a fall in GH and IGF-I levels, there was a tendency for octreotide to have a greater effect and it was better tolerated. Besser and co-workers (1992) also noted that whereas only 14% of the patients had GH levels below 5 ng/ml after bromocriptine treatment, this was true for 50% of patients after octreotide treatment.

A combination of bromocriptine and octreotide has been used in a number of patients, and it has been shown that combined treatment induces a greater decrease of GH than treatment with either drug alone at the same dosage (Halse et al. 1990).

Acromegaly Due to Ectopic GHRH Secretion

Octreotide is the treatment of choice for the ectopic GHRH syndrome, unless it can be cured by surgery. So far all cases reported in the literature show that not only GH but also GHRH levels can be suppressed by infusing somatostatin or administering somatostatin analogs (Sano et al. 1991). We have personally observed two cases of ectopic GHRH syndrome in whom there was a parallel fall in the GH and GHRH levels after a single subcutaneous injection

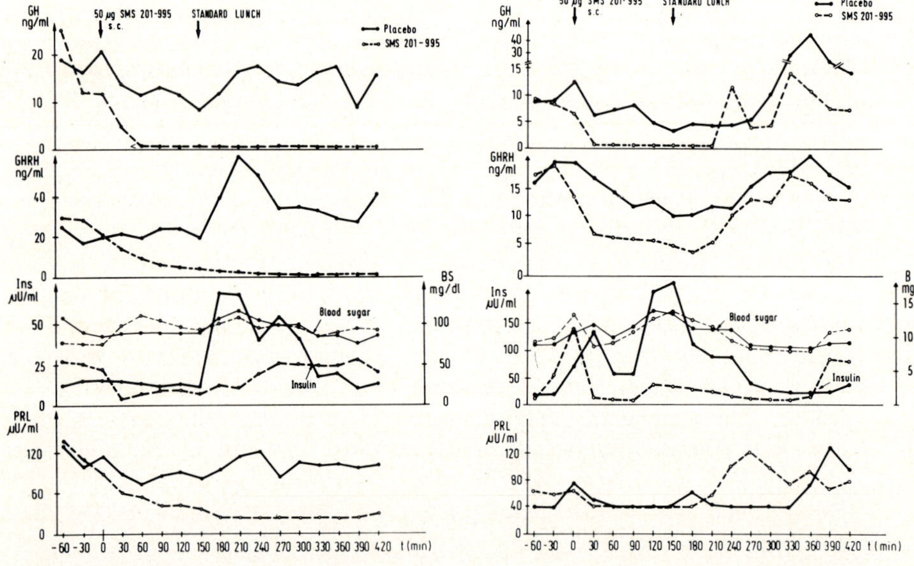

Fig. 5. GH, GHRH, insulin and PRL-levels in two female patients with an ectopic GHRH syndrome. One patient was a 14-year-old girl with a gut GHRH-producing tumor and gigantism (*left*). The other patient, a 54-year-old female, with acromegaly and an intrathoracic carcinoid tumor (*right*). Both patients had disseminated disease and both responded with a fall in GH and GHRH levels and suppression of the postprandial insulin rise after subcutaneous administration of 50 µg octreotide (SMS 201-995). The blood sugar levels are not influenced by octreotide despite insulin suppression, which is explained by the concomitant suppression of insulin antagonistic GH levels. (von Werder et al. 1988)

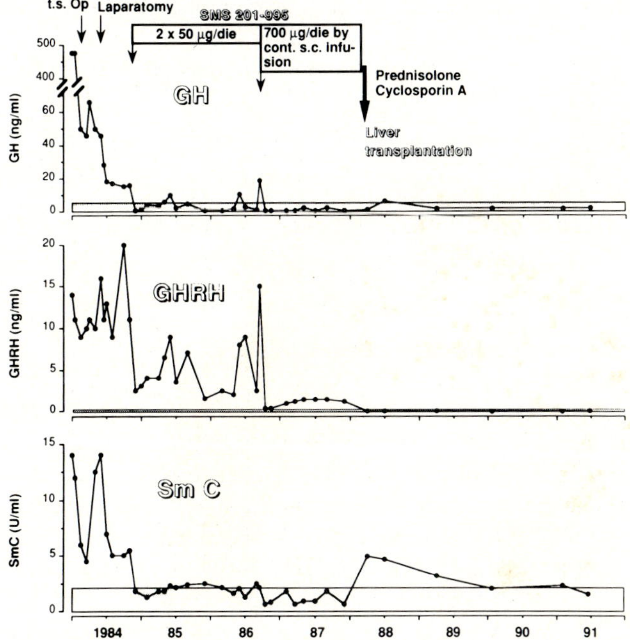

Fig. 6. GH, GHRH and Somatomedin C (*SmC*) levels in a female patient with gigantism due to an ectopic GHRH syndrome (jejunal carcinoid with liver metastases). After initial pituitary surgery (somatotroph hyperplasia extending above the sella turcica) and laparotomy followed palliative treatment with octreotide (SMS 201-995). Curative treatment with liver transplantation was performed 3 years ago. Ever since, GHGH levels have been undetectable. (von Werder et al. 1988)

of 50 µg octreotide (Fig. 5). In one patient with metastasizing liver disease originating from a jejunal carcinoid tumor, octreotide treatment lasting for over more than 4 years not only led to effective suppression of GH and GHRH levels but also to a reduction in the GHRH tumor content (von Werder et al. 1988). This young girl, who after 4 years of octreotide treatment was free of extrahepatic tumor tissue later underwent liver transplantation (Fig. 6). She has now been free of GHRH producing tumor for 4 years and her regulation of GH secretion is completely normal.

TSH-Secreting Adenomas

TSH secreting adenomas are rare, representing less than 1% of all pituitary adenomas in larger pituitary series (Beckers et al. 1991). They lead to inappropriately elevated TSH levels and may cause hyperthyroidism (Horn et al. 1976). The latter is often attributed to other causes, and the diagnosis of the pituitary tumour is, therefore, delayed until the tumor causes visual disturbances or other neurological deficits due to invasive and suprasellar tumor growth. These tumours are, therefore, difficult to operate on, and surgical removal is usually incomplete. Even after additional pituitary irradiation, only 40% of patients have normal TSH levels (Beckers et al. 1991).

Somatostatin causes inhibition of TSH secretion in normal subjects (Siler et al. 1974; Reichlin 1983) and in patients with TSH secreting tumors (Comi et al. 1987; Reschini et al. 1976). For this reason, octreotide has been introduced into the treatment of TSH-secreting adenomas. The results of octreotide therapy in 37 patients with TSH-secreting adenomas from various centers all over the world have been recently reviewed (Chanson and Warnet 1992). Twenty-one patients received an acute bolus injection of 50 or 100 μg octreotide which led to a fall in the TSH-levels in all but one patient, the nadir occurring between 3 and 6 h after octreotide injection. In ten patients α-subunit levels were also measured, which decreased in seven parallel to the TSH levels.

In 23 patients octreotide was administered at a dosage of 50 or 100 μg 2 or 3 times daily for 1 or 2 weeks. TSH levels fell and were normalized during octreotide treatment in more than 70% of the patients. Furthermore, thyroid hormone levels decreased in all and normalized in 78% of the patients with TSH-secreting adenomas. There was no difference in TSH suppression as a response to octreotide in pure TSH-secreting adenomas and mixed pituitary adenomas which in addition to α-subunits secreted either PRL or GH.

Fourteen patients were treated for more than 3 months with dosages ranging between 200 and 1500 μg octreotide/day. Only one patient was partially resistant and remained thyrotoxic during octreotide treatment, although a fall in the TSH levels was observed (Chanson and Warnet 1992). Two patients showed a later reincrease in TSH levels, despite continuous octreotide treatment.

Reduction in tumour volume was observed in five of the 14 patients, with a remarkable improvement of visual field defects in two of them (Chanson and Warnet 1992; Guillausseau et al. 1987). Side effects were comparable to those seen in acromegaly patients, i.e., two of the 14 patients developed gallstones which disappeared in one after 4 months of combined therapy with ursodeoxycholic acid (Chanson and Warnet 1992).

In summary, octreotide represents an effective medical therapy in most patients with TSH-secreting adenomas who are not cured by neurosurgery or radiotherapy. The fact that in some patients treated with octreotide TSH levels remain elevated but thyroid hormone levels become normalized raises the additional interesting possibility that octreotide has also an effect on TSH bioactivity. Octreotide may, therefore, be considered as a medical treatment of choice in TSH-secreting adenomas when previous surgery and radiotherapy have not led to cure.

Pituitary Resistance to Thyroid Hormones

Inappropriate secretion of TSH causing hyperthyroidism can be due either to TSH-secreting adenomas or to selective pituitary resistance to thyroid hormone action (PRTH) (Weintraub et al. 1981). The ideal treatment of thyroid hyperfunction should aim to reduce TSH secretion, since therapy directed against the thyroid gland would invariably result in increased TSH secretion, often in the recurrence of goiter and hyperthyroidism, and possibly in pituitary tumour expansion in the case of TSH-secreting adenomas or progress of thyrotroph hyperplasia to tumor in PRTH. The role of octreotide in TSH-secreting adenomas is already well-established (as described above). In contrast there are very few studies concerning the use of octreotide in PRTH. Beck-Peccoz et al. (1989) reported on three hyperthyroid patients with PRTH and four patients with TSH-secreting adenomas who were all briefly treated with 3×100 μg octreotide for 5 days. This regimen lowered serum TSH levels by 47% in PRTH patients, far less than in those with TSH-secreting adenomas (88%). Thyroid hormone levels were normalized only in one of the PRTH patients, whereas normalization occurred in all TSH-secreting adenoma patients. In two patients with PRTH, octreotide treatment was carried out for 6 weeks, but an escape occurred after only a few weeks in both cases. In contrast in none of the patients with TSH-secreting adenomas who underwent treatment for 1–7 months was any escape of TSH suppression from octreotide treatment observed. On the other hand, Chan et al. (1990) reported one patient with PRTH in whom octreotide had long-term beneficial effects.

Although more patients treated with higher dosages of octreotide should be studied before a definite conclusion is drawn, it appears from the present data that, unlike in TSH-secreting adenoma patients, octreotide improves hyperthyroidism in patients with PRTH in only a transient manner. This difference may be explained by the fact that in the latter situation we are dealing with a very dominant negative feedback system, the most powerful regulatory mechanism of TSH secretion (Weintraub et al. 1981). It is reasonable to assume that the fall in circulating thyroid hormones which follows the initial reduction in TSH levels induced by octreotide later elicit a reactive increase in TSH secretion that overcomes octreotide's inhibitory effect.

Nonfunctioning Pituitary Adenomas

In the absence of any hypersecretory symptoms, nonfunctioning pituitary adenomas (NFPA) usually come to medical attention only when the tumor has grown large enough to cause mass symptoms and/or secretory defects. Surgery is not curative in most patients and, in spite of additional radiotherapy, the recurrence rate is quite high, accounting for 30%–50% in different series. This has prompted the search for medical treatment using either DA agonists or gonadotropin-releasing hormone superagonists (Liuzzi et al. 1991). However, treatment with these agents has resulted in tumor shrinkage in less than ¼ of

Table 2. Effects of octreotide on tumor size in nonfunctioning pituitary adenomas

Author	Patients (n)	Dose (μg/day)	Duration (mo)	Tumor volume		
				Reduced	Same	Increased
Muhr et al. (1988)	4	150–600	0.5–1	2	2	0
Vos et al. (1988)	1	200	1.5	0	1	0
Sassolas et al. (1988)	1	200	14	1	0	0
Renard et al. (1990)	7	200	1	0	7	0
Petrini et al. (1990)	7	300	3–6	0	0	0
Warnet (1990)	22	?	1–7	2	20	0
Liuzzi et al. (1991)	20	300–500	4–10	3	14	3

the patients reported. Octreotide treatment has been recently introduced, but tumor shrinkage has been reported in only 13% (8 out of 62) patients with NFPA (Liuzzi et al. 1991; von Werder and Faglia 1992), while some patients show tumor expansion (Table 2). However, none of the patients treated so far was preselected for the presence of somatostatin receptors.

With the use of in vivo scintigraphy with radioiodinated Tyr^3-octreotide, Faglia et al. (1991) were able to show somatostatin receptors in two tumours out of 11 examined. They treated two patients shown to be positive and two patients shown to be negative on Octreoscan with octreotide. No change in tumor size occurred after 1 year treatment in patients with negative Octreoscans, while in one of those with positive somatostatin receptors a 10% reduction in tumor volume was observed within 6 months. In the other patient, an expansion of the tumor by 33% was seen within 6 months during octreotide treatment. In this patient, octreotide was stopped and the patient underwent surgery. The excised tumor showed diffuse, necrotic, and colliquative changes. Although the occurrence of spontaneous changes cannot be ruled out, it is tempting to speculate that octreotide was active in this patient, too, although in a clinically unfavorable manner. In vitro binding studies carried out on solid specimens from the tumor demonstrated a high number of somatostatin receptors similar to those observed in GH-secreting tumors, whereas no somatostatin receptors in vitro could be detected in four tumors taken from patients with negative Octreoscans (Faglia et al. 1991).

In conclusion, although pituitary scintigraphy seems to be a valid tool for screening patients, regardless of whether they have NFPAs that are somatostatin receptor positive or ones that are negative, octreotide treatment should be carefully monitored after a possible increase in tumor mass. Whether presurgical octreotide treatment may facilitate a more radical surgery of NFPA as it seems to be the case in acromegaly is an open question.

Cushing's Disease

Somatostatin has been shown to inhibit ACTH secretion from the mouse tumour cell line AtT20 and is effective in suppressing the ACTH release stimulated by ACTH-releasing hormone (CRH) from rat anterior pituitary cells in the absence of cortisol (Stalla et al. 1989). However, in a study of four patients with Cushing's disease and ACTH-producing microadenomas, treatment with octreotide of a dosage of 300–600 μg/day was only partially successful, leading to normalization of ACTH and cortisol levels in two patients (Lorcy et al. 1989). Lamberts et al. (1989) treated three patients with Nelson's syndrome. Two patients received a single dose of 200 μg octreotide and there was a subsequent reduction of ACTH from 319 and 178 pmol/l to 11.9 and 64 pmol/l 4 and 2 h after injection, respectively. The third patient received 100 μg octreotide 3 times/day for 3 days and this led to a significant decrease in the ACTH level and normalization of visual field defects and visual acuity within 6 weeks after starting therapy. However, octreotide did not affect ACTH or cortisol levels in three patients with untreated Cushing's disease. Since transsphenoidal surgery is the treatment of choice in eutopic ACTH-dependent hypercortisolism followed by radiotherapy or adrenolytical treatment, which is usually effective, no greater number of patients treated with octreotide for Cushing's disease have been investigated. From the scattered cases reported it can be deduced, however, that octreotide is not an important drug for treating pituitary ACTH-dependent hypercortisolism. However, octreotide may be very useful in the management of ectopic ACTH secretion, which also leads to bilateral adrenal hyperplasia.

Ectopic ACTH Syndrome

Although the GHRH syndrome has so far always been responsive to octreotide, this has not been the case in the ectopic ACTH and CRH syndromes (Müller and von Werder 1992). However, it has been shown that, in contrast to cases of eutopic pituitary ACTH hypersecretion, octreotide may be quite valuable in selected cases of ectopic ACTH hypersecretion. Thus, numerous single observations have been reported showing the efficacy of octreotide in suppressing ectopic ACTH secretion (Bertagna et al. 1989; Müller and von Werder 1992).

Occasionally, the ACTH inhibition induced by octreotide is so pronounced that patients experience adrenal failure necessitating cortisol substitutional therapy (Müller and von Werder 1992).

In summary, it can be concluded that octreotide is a useful tool in patients with ectopic ACTH syndrome in whom the ACTH producing tumor, which is usually malignant, cannot be surgically cured. In those patients whose response to octreotide treatment is normalization of ACTH secretion, the quality of life can be considerably improved. Patients with an extremely rare ectopic CRH syndrome leading to secondary eutopic ACTH secretion may also respond to octreotide administration, although in none of the cases mentioned has the efficacy of octreotide in directly inhibiting CRH secretion ever been shown (Müller and von Werder 1992).

PRL- and Gonadotropin Secreting Adenomas

PRL-secreting adenomas (prolactinomas) are the most common pituitary tumors in man. They respond almost unequivocally to DA agonists, which lead to inhibition of PRL secretion as well as tumor shrinkage (Bevan et al. 1992). Somatostatin, in contrast, has little effect on elevated PRL levels in patients with prolactinomas. For this reason, octreotide treatment has not been investigated in an appreciable number of patients with prolactinomas.

In contrast to prolactinomas, gonadotropin-secreting adenomas are extremely rare. These adenomas similar to TSH-producing tumours usually show suprasellar extension and grow invasively into the base of the skull. Surgical therapy is not very effective.

However, information on the effectiveness of octreotide treatment in this situation is scarce (Warnet 1992). Data are available in five patients which suggest that octreotide treatment may have a suppressive effect in ¼ of patients with gonadotropin-secreting adenomas.

Conclusion

Octreotide treatment is effective in suppressing the hormone hypersecretion caused by pituitary adenomas that is normally under physiological inhibitory control by somatostatin. Thus, the success of octreotide treatment in acromegaly and TSH producing tumors is well-established. In contrast, only individual patients with NFPAs, or ACTH- or gonadotropin-secreting tumours respond favorably to octreotide treatment, whereas prolactinomas are generally totally unresponsive.

References

Barkan AL, Kelch RP, Hopwood NJ, Beitins IZ (1988) Treatment of acromegaly with the long-acting Somatostatin analog SMS 201-995. J Clin Endocrinol Metab 66:16–23

Bauer W, Briner U, Doepfner W, Haller R, Huguenin R, Marbach P et al (1982) SMS 201-995: a very potent and selective octapeptide analogue of somatostatin with prolonged action. Life Sci 31:133–140

Beckers A, Abs R, Mahler C, Vandalem JL, Pirens G, Hennen G, Stevenaert A (1991) Thyrotropin secreting pituitary adenomas: Report of seven cases. J Clin Endocrinol Metab 72:477–483

Beck-Peccoz P, Mariotti S, Guillauseau PJ, Medri G, Piscitelli G, Bertoli A, Barbarino A, Rondena M, Chanson Ph, Pinchera A, Faglia G (1989) Treatment of hyperthyroidism due to inappropriate secretion of thyrotropin with the somatostatin analogue SMS 201-995. J Clin Endocrinol Metab 68:208–214

Bertagna X, Favrod-Coune C, Escourolle H et al (1989) Suppression of ectopic adrenocorticotropin secretion by the long-acting somatostatin analogue octreotide. J Clin Endocrinol Metab 68:988–991

Besser GM (1992) In: Liuzzi A, Sobrinho LG, Besser GM (eds) Proceedings of the Workshop "Practical Approaches to the Diagnosis and Treatment of Acromegaly". Metabolism 41 [Suppl 2]:87–90

Besser GM, Wass JAH (1987) The use of dopamine agonists in the management of acromegaly. In: Robbins RJ, Melmed S (eds) Acromegaly. Plenum, New York, pp 261–266

Bevan JS, Webster J, Burke CW, Scanlon MF (1992) Dopamine agonists and pituitary tumour shrinkage. Endocr Rev 13:220–240

Brazeau P, Vale W, Burgus R, Ling N, Butcher M, Rivier J, Guillemin R (1973) Hypothalamic polypeptide that inhibits the secretion of immunoreactive pituitary growth hormone. Science 179:77–79

Buscail L, Tauber JP, Puet-Bosquet L et al (1989) Gallstones and treatment with octreotide for acromegaly. BMJ 299:1162

Chan AW, MacFarlane IA, van Heyningen C et al (1990) Clinical hyperthyroidism due to non-neoplastic inappropriate thyrotropin secretion. Postgrad J Med 66:743–746

Chanson P, Warnet A (1992) Treatment of thyroid-stimulating hormone-secreting adenomas with octreotide. Metabolism 41 [Suppl 2]:62–65

Chiodini PG, Attanasio R, Orlandi P, Cozzi R (1991) Growth hormone release inhibiting hormone. In: Motta M (ed) Brain endocrinology, 2nd edn. Raven, New York, pp 301–313

Chiodini PG, Cozzi R, Dallabonzana D, Oppizzi G, Verde G, Petrocini M, Liuzzi A, del Pozo E (1987) Medical treatment of acromegaly with SMS 201-995, a somatostatin analogue: a comparison with bromocriptine. J Clin Endocrinol Metab 64:447–453

Ching LJC, Sandler LM, Kraenzlin ME, Burrin JM, Joplin GF, Bloom SR (1985) Long term treatment of acromegaly with a long-acting analogue of somatostatin. BMJ 290:284–287

Christensen SE, Weeke J, Orskov H, Moller N, Flyvbjerg A, Harris AG, Lund E, Jorgensen J (1987) Continuous subcutaneous pump infusions of somatostatin analogue 201–995 versus subcutaneous injection schedule in acromegalic patients. Clin Endocrinol 27:297–306

Chrubasik J, Meynadier J, Blond S et al. (1984) Somatostatin: a potent analgesic. Lancet 2:1208–1209

Comi RJ, Gesundheit N, Murray L, Gorden P, Weintraub BD (1987) Response of thyrotropin-secreting pituitary adenomas to a long-acting somatostatin analogue. N Engl J Med 317:12–17

Dowling RH, Hussaini SH, Murphy GM, Besser GM, Wass JAH (1992) Gallstones during octreotide therapy. Metabolism 41 [Suppl 2]:22–33

Ezzat S, Ren S-G, Braunstein GD, Melmed S (1992) Octreotide stimulates Insulin-like growth factor binding protein-1: a potential pituitary independent mechanism for drug action. J Clin Endocrinol Metab 75:1459–1463

Faglia G, Bazzoni N, Spada A, Arosio M, Ambrosi B, Spinelli F, Sara R, Bonino C, Lunghi F (1991) In vivo detection of somatostatin receptors in patients with functionless pituitary adenomas by means of a radioiodinated analogue of somatostatin (^{123}SDZ 204-090). J Clin Endocrinol Metab 73:580–856

Guillausseau PJ, Chanson P, Timsit J et al (1987) Visual improvement with SMS 201-995 in a patient with a thyrotropin-secreting adenoma. N Engl J Med 317:53–54

Halse J, Harris AG, Kvistborg A, Kjartansson O, Smiseth O, Djosland O, Hass G, Jervell J (1990) A randomized study of SMS 201-995 versus bromocriptine treatment in acromegaly: clinical and biochemical effects. J Clin Endocrinol Metab 70:1254–1261

Harris A (1991) Acromegaly. Sandoz, Basel

Harris AG, Prestele H, Herold K, Boerlin V (1988) Long-term efficacy of Sandostatin (SMS 201-995, octreotide) in 178 acromegalic patients: results from the international multicenter acromegaly study group. In: Lamberts SWJ (eds) Sandostatin in the treatment of acromegaly. Springer, Berlin, Heidelberg New York, pp 117–125

Heron L, Thomas F, Ruiz JM, Henan S, Schatz B, Kuhn JM (1992) Treatment of acromegaly with a longacting formulation of the somatostatin analogue laureotide. One year follow up. Abstract 714, Endocrine Society San Antonio, Texas

Hofland LJ, van Koetsveld PM, van Vroonhoven CCJ, Stefanko SZ, Lamberts SWJ (1989) Heterogeneity of growth hormone (GH) release by individual pituitary adenoma cells from acromegalic patients, as determined by the reverse hemolytic plaque assay: effects of SMS 201-995, GH-releasing hormone and thyrotropin releasing hormone. J Clin Endocrinol Metab 68:613–620

Horn K, Erhardt F, Fahlbusch R, Pickardt CR, von Werder K, Scriba PC (1976) Recurrent thyrotoxic goiter and galactorrhea-amenorrhea syndrome due to an autonomous thyrotropin and prolactin producing pituitary adenoma. J Clin Endocrinol 43:142

James R, Chatterjee S, White MC, Hall K, Moller N, Kendall-Taylor P (1989) Continuous infusion of octreotide in acromegaly. Lancet 2:1083–1087

Krulich I, Dhariwal APS, McCann SM (1968) Stimulatory and inhibitory effects of purified hypothalamic extracts on growth hormone release from rat pituitary in vitro. Endocrinology 83:783–790

Lamberts SWJ, Bakker WM, Reubi JC (1990) The value of somatostatin receptor imaging in the localization of endocrine and brain tumours. N Engl J Med 323:1246–1249

Lamberts SWJ, Uitterlinden P, Verschoor L, van Dorgen KJ, del Pozo E (1985) Longterm treatment of acromegaly with the somatostatin analogue SMS 201-995. N Engl J Med 313:1576–1580

Lamberts SWJ, Zweens M, Klijn JGM, van Vroohoven CCJ, Stefanko SZ, del Pozo E (1986) The sensitivity of growth hormone and prolactin secretion to the somatostatin analogue SMS 201-995 in patients with prolactinomas and acromegaly. Clin Endocrinol 25:201–212

Lamberts SWJ, Uitterlinden P, del Pozo E (1987) SMS 201-995 induces a continuous decline in circulating growth hormone and somatomedin-C levels during therapy of acromegalic patients for over two years. J Clin Endocrinol Metab 65:703–710

Lamberts SWJ, Uitterlinden P, Schujff PC, Klijn JGM (1988) Therapy of acromegaly with Sandostatin: the predictive value of an acute test, the value of serum somatomedin C measurements in dose adjustment and the definition of a biochemical 'cure'. Clin Endocrinol (Oxf) 289:411–420

Lamberts SWJ, Uitterlinden P, Klijn JMG (1989) The effect of the longacting somatostatin analogue SMS 201-995 on ACTH secretion in Nelson's Syndrome and Cushing's Syndrome. Acta Endocrinol 120:760–766

Liuzzi A, Chiodini PG, Botalla L, Cremascoli G, Müller EE, Silvestrini F (1974) Decrease of plasma growth hormone (GH) levels in acromegalics following CB 1542 Br alpha-ergocryptine) administration. J Clin Endocrinol Metab 38:910–912

Liuzzi A, Dallabonzana D, Oppizzi G, Cozzi R, Strada S, Arrigoni GL, Chiodini PG (1991) Is there a real medical treatment for the "non-secreting" pituitary adenomas? In: Faglia G, Beck-Peccoz P, Ambrosi B, Travaglini P, Spada A (eds) Pituitary adenomas: new trends in basic and clinical research. ICS 961, Elsevier, Amsterdam, pp 383–390

Losa M, Oeckler B, Schopohl J, Müller OA, Alba-Lopez J, von Werder K (1989) Evaluation of selective transsphenoidal adenomectomy by endocrinological testing and somatomedin-C measurement in acromegaly. J Neurosurg 70:561–567

Lorcy Y, Delambre C, Leguerrier AM et al (1989) Traitement de la maladie de Cushing par un analogue de la somatostatine (SMS 201-995): Quatres observations. Ann Endocrinol 50:311 (Abstr 106)

Mehltretter G, Heinz S, Schopohl J, von Werder K, Müller OA (1991) Long-term treatment with SMS 201-995 in resistant acromegaly: effectiveness of high doses and continuous subcutaneous infusion. Klin Wochenschr 69:83–90

Müller OA, von Werder K (1992) Ectopic production of ACTH and corticotropin-releasing hormone (CRH). J Steroid Biochem Mol Biol 43: No. 5, 403–408

Muhr C, Bergström M, Lundberg PO, Bergström K, Langström B (1988) Positron emission tomography for the in vivo characterization and follow-up of treatment in pituitary adenomas. Adv Biosci 69:163–170

Petrini L, Pilosu R, Marcello A, Mastio F, Bartolomei MP, Nardi M, Martino E (1990) Effect of octreotide (SMS 201-995) administration on the size of nonfunctional pituitary tumours. J Endocrinol Invest 13 [Suppl 1]:161

Pieters GFFM, Van Liessum PA, Smals AGH et al (1987) Longterm treatment of acromegaly with Sandostatin (SMS 201-995). Normalization of most anomalous growth hormone responses. Acta Endocrinol [Suppl] 18:9–18

Plöckinger V, Dienemann D, Quabbe H-J (19990) Gastrointestinal side-effects of octreotide during long-term treatment of acromegaly. J Clin Endocrinol Metab 71:1658–1662

Quabbe HJ (1982) Treatment of acromegaly by transsphenoidal operation, 90-yttrium implantation and bromocriptine: results in 230 patients. Clin Endocrinol (Oxf) 16:107–119

Quabbe HJ, Plöckinger U (1989) Dose-response study and long-term effect of the somatostatin analogue octreotide in patients with therapy-resistant acromegaly. J Clin Endocrinol Metab 68:873–881

Reichlin S (1983) Somatostatin. N Engl J Med 309:1495–1501, 1536–1563

Renard E, Barjon JN, Bringer J, Frèrebeau P, Jaffiol C (1990) Quick improvement of visual field complications due to extensive nonfunctioning hypothalamic or pituitary tumours with a somatostatin analogue (SMS 201-995). J Endocrinol Invest 13 [Suppl 2]:74

Reschini E, Giustina G, Cantalamessa L, Peracchi M (1976) Hyperthyroidism with elevated plasma TSH levels and pituitary tumor: Study with somatostatin. J Clin Endocrinol Metab 43:924–927

Reubi JC, Landolt AM (1989) The growth hormone responses to octreotide in acromegaly correlate with adenoma somatostatin receptor status. J Clin Endocrinol Metab 68:844–850

Reubi JC, Heitz PU, Landolt AM (1987) Visualization of somatostatin receptors and correlation with immunoreactive growth hormone and prolactin in human pituitary adenomas: evidence for different tumor subclasses. J Clin Endocrinol Metab 65:65–73

Ross DA, Wilson CB (1988) Results of transsphenoidal microsurgery for growth hormone secreting pituitary adenomas in a series of 214 patients. J Neurosurg 68:854–867

Sano T, Asa SL, Kovacs K (1991) Growth hormone releasing hormone producing tumours: clinical, biochemical and morphological manifestations. Endocr Rev 9:357–373

Sassolas G (1992) The role of sandostatins in acromegaly. Metabolism 41 [Suppl 2]:39–43

Sassolas G, Melmed S (1992) Symposium: basic somatostatin research. Metabolism 41 [Suppl 2]:11–16

Sassolas G, Serusclat P, Claustrat B, Trouillas J, Merabt S, Cohen R, Souquet JC (1988) Plasma alpha-subunit levels during the treatment of pituitary adenomas with the somatostatin analogue SMS 201-995. Horm Res 29:124–128

Sassolas G, Harris AG, James-Deidier A (1990) Long term effect of incremental doses of the Somatostatin analogue SMS 201-995 in 58 acromegalic patients. J Clin Endocrinol Metab 71:391–397

Schopohl J, Wiedemann Y, Nass R, Strasburger A, Moyto J, Garzon F, Thomas F (1993) Treatment of resistant acromegaly: high dose octreotide therapy versus a slow release formulation of the somatostatin analogue lanreotide. Exper Clin Endocr (in press)

Siler TM, Yen SSC, Vale W, Guillemin R (1974) Inhibition by somatostatin of the release of TSH induced in man by thyrotropin-releasing factor. J Clin Endocrinol Metab 38:742–746

Stalla GK, Stalla J, Mojito J, Höllt V, Oeckler R, Buchfelder M, Müller OA (1989) Regulation of corticotroph adenoma cells in vitro. Acta Endocrinol 190 [Suppl 1]:209

Stevenaert A, Harris AG, Kovacs K, Beckers A (1992) Presurgical octreotide treatment in acromegaly. Metabolism 41 [Suppl 2]:51–58

Vance ML, Harris AG (1991) Longterm treatment of 189 acromegalic patients with the somatostatin analogue octreotide. Arch Intern Med 151:1573–1578

Vos P, Croughs RJM, Thijssen JHH, van't Verlaat JW, van Ginkel LA (1988) Response of luteinizing hormone-secreting pituitary adenomas to a long-acting somatostatin analogue. Acta Endocrinol 118:587–590

Warnet A (1990) Effect of Sandostatin on optic chiasm compression due to non GH-, non TSH-secreting pituitary adenomas. J Endocrinol Invest 13 [Suppl 2]:74

Warnet A (1992) The Role of octreotide (Sandostatin) in Non-Growth Hormone-, Non-Thyroid-Stimulating Hormone-, and Non-Prolactin-Secreting Adenomas. Metabolism 41 [Suppl 2]:59–61

Weintraub BD, Gershengorn MC, Kourides IA, Fein H (1981) Inappropriate secretion of thyroid-stimulating hormone. Ann Intern Med 95:339–351

von Werder K (1975) Wachstumshormon- und Prolaktin-Sekretion des Menschen. Urban and Schwarzenberg, Munich

von Werder K, Faglia G (1992) Potential indications for octreotide in endocrinology. Metabolism 41 [Suppl 2]:91–98

von Werder K, Fahlbusch R, Losa M, Oeckler R, Pichl J, Schopohl J (1987) Decision analysis of treatment options in acromegaly. In: Robbins RJ, Melmed S (eds) Acromegaly. Plenum, New York, pp 267–280

von Werder K, Schopohl J, Wolfram G, Mojto J, Stalla GK, Losa M, Müller OA (1988) Ectopic production of pituitary hormones and releasing hormones. Adv Biosci 69:87–95

Effects of Sandostatin on Neuroendocrine Tumours of the Gastrointestinal System

K. D. Buchanan

Department of Medicine, Institute of Clinical Science, The Queen's University of Belfast, Grosvenor Road, Belfast BT12 68J, Northern Ireland

Before reviewing the effects of Sandostatin on neuroendocrine tumours (NETs) of the gastrointestinal system, it is pertinent to briefly review the clinical features of patients with such tumours.

Clinical Features

Patients with NETs may suffer from the effects of the tumour growth or from an endocrine syndrome or both. Some NETs are non-metastatic at presentation and theoretically are resectable. However, a variable number of patients with NETs may present with surgically incurable metastases, or develop such metastases later in their illness. It is in this latter group that an alternative management to surgery must be sought (Table 1). The use of Sandostatin will be mainly confined to this group.

Another feature of NETs is that they frequently grow slowly, and despite in some cases having extensive metastases, a surprisingly good quality of life can be maintained, frequently for several years (Buchanan et al. 1986b). If symptoms can be improved by a drug such as Sandostatin then the quality of life can be much better. With such slow-growing tumours which often grow to enormous size, spontaneous necrosis of tumours can result giving apparent remissions, a point which must be taken into consideration when assessing the

Table 1. Number and percentage of metastasizing neuroendocrine tumours. (From Watson et al. 1989)

	n	%		*n*	%
VIPomas	5	100	Somatostatinomas	2	50
Glucagonoma	2	100	Lung carcinoids	28	21
Mid-gut carcinoids	55	65	Insulinomas	23	13
Gastrinoma	13	54	Appendiceal carcinoids	195	3

Recent Results in Cancer Research, Vol. 129

effect of a drug on tumour growth. The indications for Sandostatin therapy in NETs are as follows:

1. The control of the endocrine syndrome. This may be in the short-term in controlling a syndrome in an operable tumour prior and during surgery, or long-term in patients with inoperable metastatic disease.
2. Anti-tumour effect.
3. In imaging of tumours and assessment of Sandostatin receptor status of NETs.

The different endocrine syndromes will be reviewed with an assessment of the role of Sandostatin in each of these. The uses of Sandostatin in the short term to prevent or treat 'endocrine crisis' that may occur during anaesthetic or surgical procedures will be discussed. The use of labelled preparations of octreotide to image tumours and to assess receptor status will be presented. Finally the potential of octreotide as an anti-tumour agent will be discussed.

The VIPoma Syndrome

VIPomas are rare tumours, the annual incidence being estimated as 0.012 per 100000 of the population (Watson et al. 1989). The syndrome was first described by Verner and Morrison in 1958. The tumours are usually pancreatic islet cell in origin and have frequently metastasized at presentation. Neuroblastomas and ganglioneuromas may also present with the syndrome. The syndrome is mediated by vasoactive intestinal polypeptide (VIP) although the tumours also secrete peptide histidine methionine (PHM).

The classical features are *w*atery *d*iarrhoea, *h*ypokalaemia, and *a*chlorhydria, which abbreviates to the acronym WDHA.

Patients present with severe watery diarrhoea, which is described as 'milky tea' and odourless, and may lose several litres of fluid per day which are rich in potassium. The situation is life-threatening and the patient can become severely dehydrated. The hypokalaemia will induce muscle weakness and even paralysis. Hepatomegaly due to tumour metastases may be present, and investigations will reveal a pancreatic tumour with hepatic metastases. At this point clinicians may diagnose an exocrine cancer, which is inoperable in a severely ill patient and not proceed to further investigation. The diagnosis is clinched by finding an elevated circulating level of VIP, and histological proof of an NET.

In the author's own experience, in six patients with the syndrome, four responded to Sandostatin. Of the two patients who did not respond, one was a baby with a ganglioneuroblastoma and the other a middle-aged woman with a metastastic VIPoma. Such remissions are confirmed in the literature (Ch'ng et al. 1986; Maton et al. 1989). Confirmation that the drug can be life-saving comes from Wynick and Bloom (1991) who report dramatic reduction in the diarrhoea within 12–24 h of administration of the drug. Lack of responsiveness has also been noted. Ruskone et al. (1982) reported two patients who initially responded but then lapsed despite increasing doses of the drug. Williams et al. (1987) found that three out of four patients showed some escape from the drug with increasing circulating VIP levels. This would be in contrast with the author's own group where the patients either responded dramatically (four out of six) or not at all (two out of six).

The action of Sandostatin in VIPomas would appear to act by suppressing secretion of VIP from the tumour. In the author's experience suppression of VIP circulating levels are usually into the normal range (Buchanan et al. 1986a, b 1990a). Brown (1990) reports that 85% of patients respond and plasma levels of VIP decrease in about 60% of patients, but she also reports that symptomatic improvement may occur without a decrease in VIP levels, suggesting that Sandostatin may control the diarrhoea by other mechanisms, possibly by a direct effect on the gut.

Patients with VIPomas are usually remarkably sensitive to the drug and will be controlled on doses such as 50 µg twice per day subcutaneously. In one patient under the author's care, control was achieved by 50 µg once per day on alternate days. However, dosages should be increased until a response is obtained up to a maximum of 1500 µg/day (Anderson and Bloom 1986).

The variability in response to Sandostatin may be due to the Sandostatin receptor status of the tumour, although Williams and Bloom (1987) argue that other factors may be implicated including increasing tumour mass or activity. Other factors may be a selective effect of Sandostatin on different VIP molecules or PHM (Maton et al. 1986; Woods et al. 1990; Mozell et al. 1990). Other possibilities include the development of tachyphylaxis to the effect of VIP or the existence of anti-VIP receptor antibodies (Maton et al. 1986).

It can be concluded that Sandostatin can be a life-saving drug in VIPoma patients, abolishing the diarrhoea, dehydration and hypokalaemia, and giving the patient a good quality of life, despite bulky metastatic disease.

Glucagonoma Syndrome

The glucagonoma syndrome is rare, since the tumours have usually grown to massive size and metastasized to the liver before the syndrome becomes apparent. The primary tumour is pancreatic islet cell, and the syndrome has the following features:

- Islet cell tumour producing glucagon
- Necrolytic migratory erythema
- Diabetes mellitus
- Cachexia
- Giant intestinal villi with malabsorption
- Hypoaminoacidaemia
- Normochromic normocytic anaemia
- Glossitis and vulvitis
- Psychiatric features

Not all of these features are present at any one time. The most characteristic feature is the skin rash, which is painful and disturbing. The diabetes mellitus is usually non-insulin dependent, and the cachexia can be severe.

Because of the rarity of these tumours, there are few reports in the literature of their management by Sandostatin. Boden et al. (1986) report successful treatment of a patient with resultant clearance of skin rash, weight gain and improvement in circulating amino acid levels. This was associated with a suppression of circulating glucagon levels to the normal range, although no effect on the diabetes was noted.

Altimari et al. (1986) also report a single case in which again there was a dramatic response to Sandostatin with clearance of the skin rash and a marked reduction in insulin requirements. Again glucagon levels were suppressed. Ch'ng et al. (1986) report successful treatment of two glucagonomas with clearance of the rash, and improvement of the diabetes in one, but only modest suppression of hyperglucagonaemia. Maton et al. (1989) reviewed the literature on the effects of Sandostatin in glucagonoma patients. The dosage was generally 50 μg twice per day, and all patients responded with clearance of the rash and weight gain, but the effect on diabetes mellitus was variable. Plasma glucagon levels fell in nine of 12 patients, but only fell to normal levels in one. In the author's experience of the management of a severely cachectic patient with an islet tumour producing several hormones including glucagon, there was no suppression of glucagon levels and no improvement in cachexia or anaemia, although the patient did not have a skin rash.

It can be concluded that Sandostatin is an effective drug in controlling the glucagonoma syndrome, although occasional patients do not respond. The skin rash clears within a few days and weight gain is achieved. The effect on the diabetes is less spectacular.

Insulinomas

Insulinomas arise in the pancreas, and the majority do not metastasize. As they are most frequently situated in the distal pancreas, surgical cure has a high chance of success. However, metastatic and inoperable insulinomas are very difficult to manage: some respond to chemotherapy (streptozotocin) although recurrence is inevitable. The hypoglycaemia may respond to diazoxide. For this reason a novel pharmacological intervention would be of immense value.

Verschoor et al. (1986) treated three patients with insulinoma for short periods of time with Sandostatin with suppression of insulin and increased plasma glucose to hyperglycaemic levels. Similar results were noted in a single patient but the drug was more efficient when administered by constant infusion (Cervigon et al. 1987). Kung et al. (1987) reported another patient with pancreatic microadenomatosis whose hypoglycaemia was controlled by Sandostatin, and this was associated with insulin suppression. Hearn et al. (1988) noted similar success in a single patient. Stehouwer et al. (1989) addressed the problem of management of a malignant insulinoma case. Sandostatin raised blood sugar and suppressed insulin levels, and the addition of verapamil, a calcium antagonist, further raised the blood sugar. Timmer et al. (1991) have, however, reported no clinical or biochemical effect on serum glucose, insulin, C peptide or glucagon in four patients. They argue that this may be due to the absence of Sandostatin receptors on the tumours. Maton et al. (1989) have reviewed 20 patients who have received Sandostatin. In 12 of the patients, insulin was suppressed and this was associated with a rise in blood glucose. In two patients, there was no improvement in hypoglycaemic episodes, and in one the symptoms became worse, the others being unchanged or not reported.

In conclusion, Sandostatin therapy for insulinoma has a variable effect, but suppresses plasma insulin and raises blood sugar in the majority. For this reason it is worth a therapeutic trial. The majority of patients studied to date have been studied very short-term, usually prior to successful surgery. There are few longer term studies of Sandostatin on malignant tumours. Variability in action may be related to Sandostatin receptors on the tumours, but also to the fact that Sandostatin will suppress not only insulin, but other counter-regulatory hormones.

Gastrinoma

Gastrinoma or the Zollinger-Ellison syndrome can be due to either a pancreatic or extrapancreatic tumour. The common extrapancreatic sites are duodenum, and sometimes in glands adjacent to the pancreas. The hypergastrinaemia results in massive hypersecretion of acid and peptic ulceration. The medical management of the syndrome has been revolutionised by the introduction of H_2 receptor antagonist drugs and the proton pump antagonists (Collins et al. 1991). For this reason the place of additional therapy such as Sandostatin appears limited, unless Sandostatin can produce better control than other drugs, or have some additional advantage.

Ellison et al. (1986) studied ten patients with gastrinoma. In all cases, Sandostatin suppressed gastrin release and inhibited acid secretion. Sandostatin also suppressed gastrin release stimulated by secretin or calcium suggesting that the action was by post receptor mechanisms. Geelhoed et al. (1986) also reported successful management of a gastrinoma patient by Sandostatin. Bauer et al. (1989) successfully controlled a benign gastrinoma with Sandostatin but were unsuccessful with respect to a malignant gastrinoma. Mozell et al. (1990) report successful management of a patient with a malignant gastrinoma by Sandostatin, the patient being followed for a 20-month period. Maton et al. (1989) review 49 patients with gastrinoma derived from the literature and treated with Sandostatin. Many of the studies were acute and confirmed that Sandostatin suppressed gastrin release and inhibited acid secretion. Of 24 patients who received Sandostatin longer term, 14 continued to suppress gastrin and acid secretion. However, nearly all patients were also receiving H_2 receptor antagonist drugs.

In the author's experience four patients were treated short term by Sandostatin. All subjects except one responded with suppression of gastrin levels but not into the normal range. The patient who did not respond had a tumour with massive hepatic metastases and enormous circulating levels of gastrin. Another patient who presented severely ill following surgery when the diagnosis was not suspected, was unable to be controlled by a combination of intravenous ranitidine and Sandostatin but was controlled when omeprazole was added.

It would appear that the indications for the use of Sandostatin in gastrinoma are limited in the face of excellent alternative therapy although there is little doubt that Sandostatin could be a useful adjunct to therapy.

GRFomas

These are very rare islet cell tumours which produce growth hormone releasing factor (GRF) which results in growth hormone hypersecretion and acromegaly. In three patients treated, all had good symptomatic response (Von Werder et al. 1984, 1986; Ch'ng et al. 1985; Wilson et al. 1985, 1986). Circulating levels of GRF and growth hormone were suppressed but not to the normal range. It would, therefore, appear that Sandostatin is very useful in the management of these patients.

Carcinoids

The term carcinoids describes a heterogeneous group of NETs arising in many sites and are chemically characterized by producing 5-hydroxy-tryptamine and 5-hydroxy-tryptophan (Watson et al. 1989). The commonest site is the appendix, but as these tumors are usually tiny and found incidentally at surgery they will not be further discussed. Carcinoids arising in the mid-gut are the next common, and the majority of them (60% – 70%) will be metastatic to the liver and produce a clinical syndrome. Lung carcinoids are the next most common and also produce a syndrome sometimes when not metastatic. Stomach and hind-gut carcinoids will not be discussed as they are frequently clinically silent.

The classical carcinoid syndrome results in flushing and diarrhoea, but patients may also wheeze, feel weak and lose weight, have left-sided cardiac lesions, and skin rashes. They may also have marked haemodynamic disturbances with tachycardia and fluctuations of blood pressure. The syndrome is mediated by many peptides and amines, including serotonin, tachykinins, calcitonin gene-related peptide, gastrin-releasing peptide, pancreatic polypeptide, chromogranin-derived peptides, and many others. Lung carcinoids produce an atypical syndrome with additional features of salivary gland enlargement, salivation, lacrimation and facial oedema (Buchanan et al. 1990b). The precise mediators of the syndrome are not thoroughly elucidated. Patients with the carcinoid syndrome may develop a crisis where the syndrome is markedly enhanced with life-threatening haemodynamic disturbances. This frequently is precipitated by surgical procedures, a variety of drugs and intercurrent infections.

From the author's own experience in carcinoid patients (Buchanan et al. 1990b) we have found 70% of patients ($n=15$) to report that diarrhoea is better or much better following Sandostatin. Flush was improved in 58% ($n=12$) and wheeze was improved in all of a small number of subjects.

There are substantial reports in the literature of the effect of Sandostatin in carcinoid patients. Altman et al. (1989) reported cutaneous and systemic improvement in a patient with malignant carcinoid syndrome. Vinik and Moattari (1989) report improvement in 14 patients with the syndrome, improvement in diarrhoea in 83%, flushing in 100% and wheezing in 100%. This was associated with suppression of urinary 5-hydroxyindole acetic acid and circulating serotonin and neuropeptide levels. Norheim et al. (1986) report that Sandostatin can block the release of neuropeptide K during pentagastrin-induced flush, and this significantly reduces the flush. Kvols et al. (1987) found episodes of flushing and diarrhoea to be improved in 22 of 25 patients.

There is some evidence that Sandostatin will prevent and improve the features of carcinoid crisis. This life-threatening clinical condition is seen frequently in subjects with carcinoid tumours subjected to surgery. The author has had experience of several such cases. Since a regime was established of administering Sandostatin prior to, during and after surgery, no such crises have been noted. Should a crisis develop, Sandostatin appears to ameliorate the features and stabilizes blood pressure. Other case reports have documented the prompt reversal of carcinoid crisis by Sandostatin (Brabant et al. 1986; Marsh et al. 1987; Woods et al. 1990). The author would support the prophylactic use of Sandostatin in patients with carcinoid tumours undergoing chemotherapy, hepatic artery embolization and surgery (Watson et al. 1989).

Somatostatinomas

Patients with somatostatinomas present with duodenal or islet cell tumours with a clinical syndrome of diabetes mellitus, cholelithiasis and steatorrhoea. It would appear illogical to treat such patients with Sandostatin, although such an approach would not be contraindicated if the patient also had another syndrome.

Tumours Producing Multiple Hormones

Not infrequently patients present with multiple syndromes which develop during the course of the disease. Patients with multiple endocrine neoplasia 1 (MEN 1) syndrome can secrete multiple hormones from the same or different endocrine glands. Sporadic tumours may also secrete multiple hormones resulting in multiple syndromes. A patient under the care of the author presented with a metastatic gastrinoma, and during the course of the illness developed syndromes of VIPoma and insulinoma, and also secreted glucagon and pancreatic polypeptide although neither of the latter resulted in a syndrome. Secretion of adenocorticotrophic hormone (ACTH) with resulting Cushing's syndrome is sometimes encountered. One patient with Cushing's syndrome and a gastrinoma treated with Sandostatin had marked clinical and biochemical improvement in the Cushing's syndrome (Bonfils et al. 1986). Two similar patients under the author's care had no such improvement with Sandostatin.

If such patients with mixed syndromes are encountered there are no contraindications to therapy with Sandostatin, and it is expected that the patients will respond in a similar fashion as patients with a single syndrome.

Receptors

NETs have receptors to Sandostatin. Krenning et al. (1989) report localization of endocrine-related tumours with a radioiodinated analogue of somatostatin and this is reviewed by Lamberts et al. (1990). This technique has allowed the in vivo labelling and imaging of NETs. Such technology may now be applied to in vitro labelling of tumours which will lead to a better understanding of the responsiveness of tumours to Sandostatin (Reubi et al. 1992).

Anti-tumour Effects

Maton et al. (1989) have reviewed the effect of Sandostatin therapy on tumour size as assessed by computed axial tomography (CAT) scan. Of the patients with NETs and liver metastases the tumours increased in size in 20, stayed unchanged in 18, and decreased in size in eight.

There is great difficulty in assessing the data. It is unethical to establish a controlled trial with Sandostatin as the drug is clearly of value and indeed life-saving in many syndromes. Further confusion results as patients are frequently undergoing multiple other therapies including embolization, chemotherapy and surgery. Some patients with mild syndromes may not be placed on Sandostatin therapy. However, they may not act as a correct control group for symptomatic patients. The natural history of the disease is also confounding as the tumours grow very slowly and may self-necrose which may lead to remissions. It is difficult to foresee how accurate trials can be established, although a report that an overwhelming number of patients have shown tumour regression would be convincing. At present there is no irrefutable evidence that Sandostatin has an anti-tumour effect.

Summary and Conclusions

Sandostatin is a drug of immense importance in the management of NETs of the gastrointestinal tract. Its effect in some syndromes is life-saving, in particular in VIPoma.

Dramatic effects have also been reported in the glucagonoma syndrome. The quality of life is considerably improved in the carcinoid syndrome and it is potentially life-saving in carcinoid crises. The drug is effective in gastrinomas, but other therapy is more effective. Its value is controversial in insulinoma although some patients are clearly improved.

Not all patients respond and this may be related to the abundance of Sandostatin receptors on the tumour or simply to tumour bulk. There is no clear-cut evidence that Sandostatin has an anti-tumour effect in these patients.

References

Anderson J, Bloom SR (1986) Neuroendocrine tumours of the gut: long-term therapy with the somatostatin analogue SMS 201-995. Scand J Gastroenterol 21 [Suppl 119]: 115–128

Altimari AF, Bhoopalam N, O'Dorisio T, Lange CL, Sandberg L, Prinzi RA (1986) Use of a somatostatin analog (SMS 201-995) in the glucagonoma syndrome. Surgery 100 (6):989–996

Altman AR, Tschen JA, Rice L (1989) Treatment of malignant carcinoid syndrome with a long-acting somatostatin analogue. Arch Dermatol 125:394–396

Bauer FE, Hummel M, Merki HS, Schulz E, Oeder R, Marbach P (1989) Long-acting somatostatin analog controls acid and gastrin secretion in benign, but in malignant, Zollinger-Ellison syndrome. J Clin Gastroenterol 11(3):282–286

Boden G, Ryan IG, Eisenschmid BL, Shelmet JJ, Owen OE (1986) Treatment of inoperable glucagonoma with the long-acting somatostatin analogue SMS 201-995. N Engl J Med 314(26):1686–1689

Bonfils S, Ruszniewski P, Laucournet H, Costil V, Rene W, Mignon M (1986) Long-term management of Zollinger-Ellison syndrome with SMS 201-995, a long-lasting somatostatin analog. Program of the 6th International Symposium on Gastrointestinal Hormones, Vancouver, Canada, July 6–10, 1986. Can J Physiol Pharmacol, p 63

Brabant G, Muller MJ, Rotsch M et al (1986) Treatment of carcinoid syndrome and VIPoma with a long-acting somatostatin analogue (SMS 201-995). Scan J Gastroenterol 21 [Suppl 119]:117–180

Brown NJ (1990) Octreotide: a long-acting somatostatin analog. Am J Med Sci 300 (4):267–273

Buchanan KD, Shaw C, O'Hare MMT, Dalzell G (1986a) Evaluation of SMS 201-995 in gastrointestinal APUDomas. Scand J Gastroenterol 21 [Suppl 119]:199–205

Buchanan KD, Johnston CF, O'Hare MMT, Ardill JES, Shaw C, Collins JSA, Watson RGP, Atkinson AB, Hadden DR, Kennedy TL, Sloan JM (1986b) Neuroendocrine tumours – a european view. Am J Med 81 [Suppl 6B]:14–22

Buchanan KD, Collins JSA, Varghese A, Johnston CF, Shaw C (1990a) Sandostatin and the Belfast experience. Digestion 45 [Suppl 1]:11–16

Buchanan KD, Shaw C, McGrath SJ, McKillop JM, Harrison E, Johnston CF, McGuigan J, Gibbons JRP (1990b) Regulatory peptide content of lung and mid-gut carcinoid tumours. Q J Med 77 (282):1091

Cervigon PSG, Navarro JIF, de Diego JS, Asensi AC, Hernandez FC, Jara Albarran A (1987) Tratamiento preoperatorio de la hipoglucemia debida a un insulinoma con el analogo de somatostatina SMS 201-995. Med Clin (Barc) 89(12):511–513

Ch'ng JLC, Christofides ND, Kraenzlin ME, Keshavarzian A, Burrin JM, Woolf IL, Hodgson HJF, Bloom SR (1985) Growth hormone secretion dynamics in a patient with ectopic growth hormone-releasing factor production. Am J Med 79:135–138

Ch'ng JLC, Anderson JV, Williams SJ, Carr DH, Bloom SR (1986) Remission of symptoms during long term treatment of metastatic pancreatic endocrine tumours with long acting somatostatin analogue. Br Med J 292:981–982

Collins JSA, Buchanan KD, Kennedy TL, Johnston CF, Ardill JES, Sloan JM, McIlrath EM, Russel C (1991) Changing patterns in presentation and management of the Zollinger-Ellison syndrome in Northern Ireland, 1970–1988. Q J Med (New Series) 78 (287):215–225

Ellison EC, O'Dorisio TM, Sparks J, Mekhjian HS, Fromkes JJ, Woltering EA, Carey LC (1986) Observations on the effect of a somatostatin analog in the Zollinger-Ellison syndrome: implications for the treatment of APUDomas. Surgery 100(2):437

Geelhoed GW, Bass BL, Mertz SL, Becker KL (1986) Somatostatin analog: effects on hypergastrinemia and hypercalcitoninemia. Surgery 100(6):962–970

Hearn PR, Ahmed M, Woodhouse NJY (1988) The use of SMS 201-995 (somatostatin analogue) in insulinomas. Hormone Res 29:211–213

Krenning EP, Breeman WAP, Kooij PPM, Lamberts JS, Bakker WH, Koper JW, Ausema L, Reubi JC, Lamberts SWJ (1989) Localisation of endocrine-related tumours with radioiodinated analogue of somatostatin. Lancet 1:242–244

Kung AWC, Ma JTC, Wang C, Fu KH, Lam KSL, Yeung RTT, Boey J (1987) Prevention of hypoglycaemia in a patient with pancreatic microadenomatosis by a long-acting somatostatin analogue SMS 201-995. Clin Endocrinol 27:469–473

Kvols LK, Buck M, Moertel CG, Schutt AJ, Rubin J, O'Connell MJ, Hahn RG (1987) Treatment of metastatic islet cell carcinoma with a somatostatin analogue (SMS 201-995). Ann Intern Med 107:162–168

Lamberts SWJ, Bakker WH, Reubi J-C, Krenning EP (1990) Clinical application of somatostatin analogs. Part I. Metabolism 39 (9) [Suppl 2]:152–155

Marsh HM, Martin JK, Kvols LK et al (1987) Carcinoid crisis during anesthesia: successful treatment with a somatostatin analogue. Anesthesiology 66:89–91

Maton PN, O'Dorisio TM, O'Dorisio MS, Malarkey WB, Gower WJ Jr, Gardner JD, Jensen RT (1986) Successful therapy of pancreatic cholera with the long-acting somatostatin analogue SMS 201-995. Relation between plasma concentrations of drug and clinical and biochemical responses. Scand J Gastroenterol 21 [Suppl 119]:181–186

Maton PN, Gardner JD, Jensen RT (1989) Use of long-acting somatostatin analog SMS 201-995 in patients with pancreatic islet cell tumors. Dig Dis Sci 34 (3):28S–39S

Mozell E, Woltering EA, O'Dorisio TM, Fletcher WS, Sinclair AJ, Hill D (1990) Effect of somatostatin analog on peptide release and tumor growth in the Zollinger-Ellison syndrome. Surg Gynecol Obstet 170:476–484

Norheim I, Theodorsson-Norheim E, Brodin E, Oberg K (1986) Tachykinins in carcinoid tumors; their use as a tumor marker and possible role in the carcinoid flush. J Clin Endocrinol Metab 63:605

Reubi JC, Laissue J, Krenning E, Lamberts SWJ (1992) Somatostatin receptors in human cancer: incidence, characteristics, functional correlates and clinical implications. J Steroid Biochem Mol Biol 43(1–3):27–35

Ruskone A, Rene E, Chayvialle JA, Bonin N, Pignal F, Kremer M, Bonfils S, Rambaud JC (1982) Effect of somatostatin on diarrhea and on small intestinal water and electrolyte transport in a patient with pancreatic cholera. Dig Dis Sci 27:459–466

Stehouwer CDA, Lems WF, Fischer HRA, Hackeng WHL (1989) Malignant insulinoma: is combined treatment with verapamil and the long-acting somatostatin analogue octreotide (SMS 201-995) more effective than single therapy with either drug? Neth J Med 35:86–94

Timmer R, Koningsberger JC, Erkelens DW, Thijssen JHH, Lips CJM, Koppeschaar HPF (1991) No effect of the long-acting somatostatin analogue octreotide in patients with insulinoma. Neth J Med 38:199–203

Verner JV, Morrison AB (1958) Islet cell tumour and a syndrome of refractory watery diarrhea and hypokalemia. Am J Med 25:374–380

Verschoor L, Uitterlinden P, Lamberts SWJ, del Pozo E (1986) On the use of a new somatostatin analogue in the treatment of hypoglycaemia in patients with insulinoma. Clin Endocrinol 25:555–560

Vinik A, Moattari AR (1989) Use of somatostatin analog in management of carcinoid syndrome. Dig Dis Sci 34(3):14S–27S

Von Werder K, Losa M, Muller OA, Schweiberer L, Fahlbusch R, del Pozo E (1984) Treatment of metastasizing GRF-producing tumor with a long-acting somatostatin analogue. Lancet ii:282–283

Von Werder K, Losa M, Stalla GK, Muller OA, Mayr B, Schweiberer L, Fahlbusch LR (1986) Long-term treatment of a metastasizing GRFoma with a somatostatin analogue (SMS 201-995) in a girl with gigantism. Scand J Gastroenterol 21 [Suppl 119]:238–242

Watson RGP, Johnston CF, O'Hare MMT, Anderson JR, Wilson BG, Coillins JSA, Sloan JM, Buchanan KD (1989) The frequency of gastrointestinal endocrine tumours in a well-defined population – Northern Ireland 1970–1985. Quart J Med (New Series) 72 (267):647–657

Williams G, Bloom SR (1987) Long-term treatment of VIPoma and glucagonoma with Sandostatin. In: O'Dorisio TM (ed) Sandostatin in the treatment of gastroenteropancreatic endocrine tumors. Springer, Berlin Heidelberg New York

Wilson DM, Hoffman AR (1985) Reduction of pituitary size in a patient with a GRF secreting islet cell tumor by continuous infusion of a somatostatin analogue. Program of the Endocrine Society 6th Annual Meeting, Baltimore, Maryland, June 19–21, 1985, p 39

Wilson DM, Hoffman AR (1986) Reduction of pituitary size by the somatostatin analogue SMS 201-995 in a patient with an islet cell tumour secreting growth hormone releasing factor. Acta Endocrinol 113:23–28

Woods HF, Bax NDS, Ainsworth I (1990) Abdominal carcinoid tumours in Sheffield. Dig 45 [Suppl 1]:17–22

Wynick D, Bloom SR (1991) The use of the long-acting somatostatin analog octreotide in the treatment of gut neuroendocrine tumours. J Clin Endocrinol Metab 73(1):1–3

Somatostatin Analogues in the Treatment of Pancreatic Neoplasia

M.K. Müller

Medizinische Klinik IV, Gastroenterologie, Theodor-Kutzer-Ufer, W-6800 Mannheim, FRG

Acute Effects of Somatostatin: Regulation of Pancreatic Functions

Infusion of somatostatin in animals or humans exhibits an inhibitory effect on exocrine and endocrine pancreatic function, while enteral somatostatin administration inhibits interdigestive pancreatic enzyme, water, and bicarbonate output. The inhibitory effect of somatostatin on pancreatic protein secretion is significantly greater than that on water and bicarbonate secretion (Lin et al. 1983). It is likely that physiologic increases in somatostatin plasma concentrations, as they are observed in response to a meal, inhibit pancreatic enzyme output. Although the physiologic role of endogenous somatostatin in the regulation of pancreatic functions is not fully understood, the available data suggest that somatostatin may be involved in the regulation of pancreatic secretory response to a meal.

Endogenous and exogenous somatostatin also inhibit glucose-dependent insulin or glucagon secretion with glucagon being more sensitive to the action of somatostatin than insulin (Weir et al. 1980; Fujimoto et al. 1975). The inhibitory action of somatostatin on pancreatic hormone release is also considered to be of physiologic importance.

In keeping with in vivo observations, somatostatin also exhibits strong inhibitory effects on endocrine cells in vitro. However, in contrast to its strong inhibitory effects on the exocrine pancreas in vivo, somatostatin has no direct effects on it in vitro, either on isolated perfused whole pancreas or on isolated lobules or acinar preparations (Singh 1986; Müller et al. 1988 a). Thus somatostatin failed to inhibit basal or stimulated exocrine secretion in vitro, independent of species or mode of stimulation (hormonal, cholinergic). Simultaneous measurement of exocrine and endocrine pancreatic and gastric responses to somatostatin in an isolated perfused stomach-pancreas preparation demonstrated that even high concentrations of somatostatin had no effect on exocrine pancreatic secretion, while at the same time they strongly inhibited endocrine pancreatic and gastric functions (Müller et al. 1988 b). Since acinar cell receptors for somatostatin are well characterized and have been shown to

Recent Results in Cancer Research, Vol. 129

be intact even in in vitro preparations (Sakamoto et al. 1984; Singh 1986), it has been suggested that they serve functions other than direct inhibition of enzyme secretion. The marked inhibitory effects of somatostatin on acinar cell functions in vivo and the lack of effect in vitro suggest an indirect mechanism of action, such as secondary release of inhibitory peptides and/or neurotransmitters, inhibition of release of stimulatory mediators such as cholecystokinin (CCK) or acetylcholine, or a decrease in pancreatic perfusion (Schönfeld et al. 1989).

Recent data suggest that at least part of the inhibitory action of somatostatin on acinar cells may be due to the inhibition of insulin release, which has been shown to potentiate CCK- and acetylcholine-stimulated enzyme secretion (Müller et al. 1986, 1987; Lee et al. 1990).

Chronic Effects of Somatostatin

Regulation of Pancreatic Growth

In contrast to the strong inhibitory effect in acute experiments, chronic administration of somatostatin does not cause significant exocrine pancreatic insufficiency either in man or animals. Somatostatin inhibits both spontaneous, protease-inhibitor-induced and caerulein-stimulated pancreatic growth in rodents. These observations support the hypothesis that somatostatin may not only participate in the acute control of pancreatic secretion, but may also be involved in the long-term regulation of pancreatic growth and acinar enzyme synthesis (Müller et al. 1988 b; Morisset et al. 1982, 1984; Sarfati et al. 1985; Senegas-Balas et al. 1985). The inverse relationship between pancreatic somatostatin content and the acceleration of pancreatic growth supports the hypothesis that this peptide may serve as an "antigrowth factor" (Sarfati et al. 1985; Müller et al. 1988 b).

Since somatostatin inhibits pancreatic growth induced by both exogenously and endogenously released CCK, a direct action of somatostatin at the acinar cell level seems likely (Morisset et al. 1982; Müller et al. 1989). Possible other mechanisms by which somatostatin may act as an antigrowth factor are inhibition of the release of trophic peptides by hormonal pathways and also increased release into the pancreatic juice (Müller et al. 1988 b).

Inhibition of Tumor Growth

Numerous clinical studies have shown beneficial effects of somatostatin on neuroendocrine tumors. These effects are largely due to the control of peptide-induced symptoms in the treatment of vipoma and carcinoid tumors and also some other hormone-secreting tumors (Müller et al. 1992). In addition, antiproliferative actions of somatostatin on various solid tumors including tumors of the pancreas have been reported.

Approximately 95% of all pancreatic tumors occur within the exocrine portion of the pancreas. They may be derived from ductal epithelium, acinar cells, connective tissue or lymphatic deposits. The most common cancer is ductal adenocarcinoma which accounts for about 80% of all pancreatic cancers. The overall 5-year survival rate is 1%–2%. Surgical resection, which is the only available potentially curative treatment, requires a localized tumor with absence of metastasis. The operative mortality is about 5%. It is usually associated with postoperative complications such as a leak of the pancreaticojejunal anastomosis. The majority of patients with pancreatic adenocarcinoma have unresectable tumors. The predicted survival in these patients averages 4–5 months. Radiotherapy and chemotherapy offer no real advantages. Although the general resistance of pancreatic cancer cells to conventional chemotherapy is well-known, the mechanisms behind this phenomenon are not well understood.

Previously, studies on the effect of somatostatin on tumor growth were hampered by its short half-life of 1–2 min, but now the development of long-acting somatostatin analogues has made it possible to study the long-term effects of somatostatin on pancreatic tumor growth. Studies in Wistar/Lewis rats have shown somatostatin analogues to have an antiproliferative effect on the growth of the acinar pancreatic tumor DNCP-322 (Redding and Schally 1984). Treatment of Syrian golden hamsters bearing *N*-nitrosobis(2-oxopropyl)amine (BOP)-induced pancreatic carcinomas with the somatostatin analogue RC-160 and the agonist [D-Trp^6] luteinizing hormone-releasing hormone (LH-RH) showed that either substance is inhibitory, but that the combination had the strongest tumor-inhibiting effect (Szende et al. 1990).

The growth of human pancreatic cancers implanted in nude mice could be inhibited by intraperitoneal injections of 100 µg/kg SMS 201-995 three times daily for 7 weeks. The tumor growth inhibitory action of somatostatin was evident independent of whether the tumors were CCK-receptor negative (CAV) or positive (SKI) and whether treatment with somatostatin began right after transplantation or after a delay of 21 days (Upp et al. 1988). Further studies by the same group showed that somatostatin may lack an inhibitory effect on other human ductal adenocarcinomas transplanted into nude mice. It was concluded from these studies that pancreatic cancers from different patients may well respond variably to the inhibitory effects of both somatostatin and hormone receptor antagonists like tamoxifen (Poston et al. 1990). Only preliminary data exist on the effect of somatostatin analogues in humans (see also p. 13 of this volume). In a phase II trial on 14 patients with metastatic pancreatic cancer an objective antitumor effect could not be observed with 100–200 µg octreotide (Sandostatin) three times daily (Klijn et al. 1990).

In experiments on the effect of several gastrointestinal hormones on the growth of the human pancreatic cancer cell lines of ductal origin PANC-1 and MIA PaCa-2 neither CCK nor somatostatin had any demonstrable effect (Liehr et al. 1990). However, it is possible, that somatostatin exerts its inhibitory action in some tumors only in combination with other peptides because observations in MIA PaCa-2 cell cultures have shown that somatostatin alone has no effect whereas the combination of epidermal growth factor (EGF) and somatostatin resulted in a significant inhibition of EGF-induced growth (Liebow et al. 1986).

In contrast to the number of studies showing inhibition or no effect of somatostatin on pancreatic tumor growth, a recent study shows that low doses of somatostatin (5 μg/kg Sandostatin) do have a tumor-promoting effect in the Syrian golden hamster model of nitrosamine-induced pancreatic carcinogenesis (Haddock et al. 1991). An explanation for that conflicting observation could not be offered.

Mechanisms of Action of Somatostatin on Pancreatic Tumor Growth

The mechanisms of the antiproliferative effects of somatostatin are still largely speculative. One possible mechanism by which somatostatin inhibits growth of pancreatic adenocarcinomas is by inhibition of the trophic response of pancreatic cancer cells to gastrointestinal hormones like gastrin, secretin, bombesin, vasoactive intestinal polypeptide, insulin or CCK.

CCK or caerulein have indeed been reported to be trophic for some pancreatic adenocarcinomas (Lhoste et al. 1985), and high-affinity cholecystokinin receptors have been demonstrated on membrane preparations from SKI tumors (Newman et al. 1986). However, for other human pancreatic cancer cell lines of ductal origin like PANC-1 and MIA PaCa-2, only insulin and EGF but not CCK seem to be trophic factors (Liehr et al. 1990).

Another possibility would be a direct inhibitory effect of somatostatin on pancreatic cancer cells. In contrast to findings in normal acinar cells, however, somatostatin receptors could not be detected on human exocrine pancreatic adenocarcinomas obtained at surgery (Reubi et al. 1988) and consequently binding of SMS 201-995 to human pancreatic cancers could also not be observed (Srkalovic et al. 1990). Somatostatin receptors have been characterized on AR42J cells and binding of somatostatin analogues like RC-160 und RC-98-I to pancreatic cancer cell lines has been reported (Srkalovic et al. 1990). Experiments in vitro on the undifferentiated human pancreatic cancer cell line MIA PaCa-2 showed activation of dephosphorylation of the EGF receptor by somatostatin, which prevents EGF-induced growth (Hierowski et al. 1985; Liebow et al. 1986).

Conclusions

Some of the conflicting results on the effect of somatostatin on pancreatic tumor growth reported in the literature are likely to be due to the heterogeneity of pancreatic cancer, subpopulations of cell lines with different biological properties, different stages of cancer cell differentiation, different experimental models and different potency of somatostatin analogues.

Furthermore some of the conflicting observations like the tumor-promoting effect of low doses of somatostatin in the Syrian golden hamster model of nitrosamine-induced pancreatic carcinogenesis may also be due to hitherto unknown and dose-dependent actions on the part of somatostatin analogues.

Further work needs to be done with somatostatin and its analogues in both animals and humans before these peptides should be offered as a possible treatment regimen for human pancreatic cancer. The combination of somatostatin with LH-RH agonists seems to be a promising new therapeutic modality.

References

Fujimoto WY, Ensinck JW, Williams RH (1975) Somatostatin inhibits insulin and glucagon release by monolayer cell cultures of rat endocrine pancreas. Life Sci 15:1999–2004

Haddock G, Harrison DJ, Carter DC (1991) The effect of the somatostatin analogue SMS 201-995 on experimental pancreatic carcinogenesis in the Syrian golden hamster. Carcinogenesis 12:1103–1107

Hierowski MT, Liebow C, du Sapin K, Schally AV (1985) Stimulation by somatostatin of dephosphorylation of membrane proteins in pancreatic cancer MIA PaCa-2 cell line. FEBS Lett 179:252–256

Klijn JGM, Hoff AM, Planting ASTh, Verweij J, Kok T, Lamberts SWJ, Portengen H, Foekens JA (1990) Treatment of patients with metastatic pancreatic and gastrointestinal tumours with the somatostatin analogue Sandostatin: a phase II study including endocrine effects. Br J Cancer 62:627–630

Lee KY, Zhou L, Ren XS, Chang TM, Chey WY (1990) An important role of endogenous insulin on exocrine pancreatic secretion in rats. Am J Physiol 258:G268–G274

Lhoste E, Aprahamian M, Pousse A, Hoeltzel A, Stock-Damge C (1985) Combined effect of chronic bombesin and secretin or cholecystokinin on the rat pancreas. Peptides 6:83–87

Liebow C, Hierowski M, du Sapin K (1986) Hormonal control of pancreatic cancer growth. Pancreas 1:44–48

Liehr RM, Melnykovych G, Solomon TE (1990) Growth effects of regulatory peptides on human pancreatic cancer lines PANC-1 and MIA PaCa-2. Gastroenterology 98:1666–1674

Lin TM, Evans DC, Shaar CJ, Root MA (1983) Action of somatostatin on stomach, pancreas, gastric mucosa blood flow, and hormones. Am J Physiol 244:G40–G45

Morisset J, Genik P, Lord A, Solomon TE (1982) Effects of chronic administration of somatostatin on rat exocrine pancreas. Regul Pept 4:49–58

Morisset JH, Genik P, Dumont Y, Larose L (1984) Development of pancreatic function and control of pancreatic growth in an animal model. J Pediatr Gastroenterol Nutr 3 [Suppl 1]:36–42

Müller MK, Scheck T, Demol P, Goebell H (1986) Interaction of acetylcholine and gastric inhibitory polypeptide (GIP) on endocrine and exocrine rat pancreatic secretion: augmentation of acetylcholine-induced amylase and volume secretion by the insulinotropic action of gastric inhibitory polypeptide. Digestion 33:45–52

Müller MK, Scheck T, Dreesmann V, Miodonski A, Goebell H (1987) GIP potentiates CCK stimulated pancreatic enzyme secretion: correlation of anatomical structures with physiological effects. Pancreas 2:106–113

Müller MK, Kessel B, Hütt T, Layer P, Goebell H (1988 a) Effects of somatostatin-14 on gastric and pancreatic responses to hormonal and neural stimulation using an isolated perfused stomach and pancreas preparation. Pancreas 3:303–310

Müller MK, Rünzi M, Schönfeld J, Layer P, Goebell H (1988 b) Is there a physiological role for somatostatin in the pancreatic juice. Pancreas 3:609A

Müller MK, Meisse F, Roth R, Pickhardt J, Schönfeld J, Rünzi M, Goebell H (1989) Dose dependent effects of somatostatin on camostat-induced hypertrophy and hyperplasia of the pancreas. Gastroenterology 96:532A

Müller MK, Niederle N, Singer MV (1992) Neuroendokrine Tumoren des Gastrointestinaltrakts. Fortschr Med 110:24–26, 37–41

Newman JB, Lluis F, Townsend CM Jr (1986) Somatostatin. In: Thompson JC, Geeley GH Jr, Rayford PL, Townsend CM Jr (eds) Gastrointestinal endocrinology. McGraw Hill, New York, pp 286–299

Poston GJ, Townsend CM Jr, Rajaraman S, Thompson JC, Singh P (1990) Effect of somatostatin and tamoxifen on the growth of human pancreatic cancers in nude mice. Pancreas 5:151–157

Redding TW, Schally AV (1984) Inhibition of growth of pancreatic carcinomas in animal models by analogs of hypothalamic hormones. Proc Natl Acad Sci USA 81:248–252

Reubi JC, Horisberger U, Essed CE, Jeekel J, Klijn JGH, Lamberts SWJ (1988) Absence of somatostatin receptors in human exocrine pancreatic adenocarcinomas. Gastroenterology 95:760–763

Sakamoto C, Goldfine I, Williams JA (1984) The somatostatin receptor on isolated acinar cell plasma membranes. J Biol Chem 25:9623–9627

Sarfati PD, Genik P, Morisset J (1985) Caerulein and secretin induced pancreatic growth: a possible control by endogenous pancreatic somatostatin. Regul Pept 11:263–273

Schönfeld J, Müller MK, Demirtas B, Soukop J, Rünzi M, Goebell H (1989) Effect of neural blockade on somatostatin-induced inhibition of exocrine pancreatic secretion. Digestion 43:81–86

Senegas-Balas F, Balas D, Pradayrol L, Laval J, Bertrand C, Ribet A (1985) Long-term effect of somatostatin 14 on mouse, antrum, intestine and exocrine pancreas. Acta Anat 121:124–132

Singh M (1986) Effect of somatostatin on amylase secretion from in vivo and in vitro rat pancreas. Dig Dis Sci 31:506–512

Srkalovic G, Cai RZ, Schally AV (1990) Evaluation of receptors for somatostatin in various tumors using different analogs. J Clin Endocrin Metab 70:661–669

Szende B, Srkalovic G, Schally AV, Lapis K, Groot K (1990) Inhibitory effects of analogs of luteinizing hormone-releasing hormone and somatostatin on pancreatic cancers in hamsters. Cancer 65:2279–2290

Upp JR, Olson D, Poston GJ, Alexander RW, Townsend CM, Thompson JC (1988) Inhibition of growth of two human pancreatic adenocarcinomas in vivo by somatostatin analog SMS 201-995. Am J Surg 155:29–35

Weir GC, Schwarz JA, Mathe CJ (1980) Inhibition of glucagon and insulin secretion from the perfused rat pancreas by a B-cell selective somatostatin analog. Metabolism 29:68–70

Somatostatin and Somatostatin Analogues in Human Breast Carcinoma

G. Prévost [1] and L. Israel [2]

[1] Institut d'Oncologie Cellulaire et Moléculaire Humaine, 129 route de Stalingrad, 93000 Bobigny, France
[2] Service d'Oncologie Médicale, CHU Avicenne, 125 route de Stalingrad, 93000 Bobigny, France

Introduction

Somatostatin is a tetradecapeptide that was initially isolated from the hypothalamus and was found to be an inhibitor of growth hormone (GH) secretion (Brazeau et al. 1973) and, under certain conditions, of prolactin (PRL) release (Kimura et al. 1986). However, the therapeutic use of natural somatostatin is limited by its short half-life and the short duration of its antisecretory effects (Thomas et al. 1991). In order to increase the therapeutic efficacy of the drug, somatostatin analogues with a prolonged half-life have been synthesized (e.g., BIM-23014C, RC160, and SMS201-995).

GH, PRL, and various growth factors such as insulin-like growth factor I (IGF-I), epidermal growth factor (EGF), and transforming growth factor α (TGFα) are involved in the growth and malignant transformation of human breast cancer cells (McGuire et al. 1988). A decrease in plasma GH levels results in inhibition of the synthesis of IGF-I (Yee et al. 1989), and the plasma concentration of EGF is also decreased after in vivo treatment with somatostatin in patients with psoriasis (Ghirlanda et al. 1983). It is this fall in plasma GH, IGF-I, and EGF levels induced by somatostatin treatment which may partially explain the mechanism by which the drug could inhibit the growth of breast cancer cells.

In addition to their indirect action, several somatostatin analogues and the natural peptide have also been demonstrated to have growth inhibitory activities in vitro with different cell lines of human breast tumors (Setyono-Han et al. 1987; Prévost et al. 1991 a, b). Previous studies have shown specific receptors for these somatostatin analogues to be present in 15%–90% of human breast tumors (Reubi et al. 1987; Prévost et al. 1992).

Thus, the mammary tumor growth inhibition observed in nude mice after infusion of somatostatin analogues may be mediated by direct and/or endocrine/paracrine pathways (Szende et al. 1989). Furthermore, preliminary clinical studies in which somatostatin or its analogues were administered to patients with advanced breast cancer have demonstrated the drug to have

Recent Results in Cancer Research, Vol. 129

some antitumor activities without any toxic side effects (Morère et al. 1989; Vennin et al. 1989; Stolfi et al. 1990).

Experimental Data

Some somatostatin analogues inhibit both the in vivo and in vitro cell growth of human breast carcinoma (Prévost et al. 1991 a, b) and other experimental models such as prostatic carcinoma (Bogden et al. 1990) and small-cell lung carcinoma (Taylor et al. 1988).

In Vivo Effects of Somatostatin Analogues

Growth inhibition of human breast tumor xenografts (MCF-7, 13732NF, MTW9aR) by BIM-23014C (Somatuline) was found to be dose-related in the subrenal capsule assay (Prévost et al. 1992; Thomas et al. 1992). With MCF-7 solid tumor, 90% tumor size reduction was obtained after 6 days of treatment with 50 μg administered subcutaneously twice a day. This inhibitory effect was greater than a surgical bilateral ovariectomy (60%). RC160 exerted inhibitory effects on the growth of MTX mammary carcinoma (40% of tumor volume control at 25 μg per day subcutaneously for 1 month) (Szende et al. 1989). The combination of [D-Trp^{6}] – luteinizing hormone-releasing hormone (LHRH) and RC160 (10%) was more effective, and approached the effect of surgical ovariectomy (no tumor detectable).

When mice bearing MCF-7 tumors were infused with SMS201-995 (Sandostatin) (10 μg/kg per hour), tumor growth was inhibited by 98% and 85% at days 6 and 15 of the treatment, respectively (Weckbecker et al. 1990). In the same model, RC160 produced comparable effects. These results were confirmed by the study of Weber et al. (1989). SMS201-995 slowed the growth of both MCF-7 and BT20 human breast xenografts (4 and 50 μg respectively, twice a day subcutaneously) in nude mice over a period of 49 days. For MCF-7 tumors, doubling time was increased from 13.2 to 19 days.

In Vitro Effects of Somatostatin Analogues

The growth-inhibitory effects of Sandostatin and somatostatin were demonstrated on the estrogen receptor-positive cell lines (MCF-7, ZR-75) and on the estrogen receptor-negative cell line (MDAMB-436) (Nelson et al. 1989). SMS201-995 significantly reduced the MCF-7 cell growth induced by serum, estradiol, insulin, and IGF-I in both short- and long-term experiments. A bell-shaped curve response was obtained, with an optimal inhibitory effect at the concentration of 10 n*M* (Setyono-Han et al. 1987). SMS201-995 mainly exerts its effect in vitro by enhancing the rate of programmed cell death in the MCF-7 cell line (Pagliacci et al. 1991). The antiproliferative effects of somatostatin and SMS201-995 were studied with other cell lines such as CG5 (MCF-7 variant), T47D, and ZR-75-1 (Scambia et al. 1988). Both peptides (100 n*M*) markedly inhibited CG5 cell growth with a maximal inhibition of about 40% compared with control cells. The effect on T47D and ZR-75 cells was much less evident. The required presence of estradiol in culture media in order to observe SMS201-995 inhibitory effects is still controversial, and the reason for this may be clonal variations of the tested cell lines.

BIM-23014C inhibited in vitro the growth of the two steroid-dependent cell lines MCF-7 and T47D (Prévost et al. 1991 a, b). Similarly shaped curve responses were observed in the presence or absence of serum (60%–70% of cell control with 10 n*M*), indicating that no serum factors were required to obtain an inhibitory effect with the peptide. However, this inhibition is only obtained in the absence of estradiol in the media. No effect was observed with the steroid-independent cell line MDAMB-231 despite the presence of BIM-23014C receptors, indicating that their presence was not sufficient to get in vitro growth inhibition.

Somatostatin Receptor in Breast Tumor Cells

The presence of specific receptors for somatostatin on a human breast cell line (MCF-7) was first reported by Setyono-Han et al. (1987). Scatchard analysis showed a single class of high-affinity binding sites for ^{125}I-Tyr^{3}-Sandostatin with a K_d of 73 p*M* and 250 molecules per cell. Values for somatostatin receptor-positive breast tumors are variable, ranging from 15% to 90% (Reubi et al. 1987, 1990; Fekete et al. 1989; Prévost et al. 1992). This variation could be explained by differences in the visualization techniques and the labeled analogues (Murthy et al. 1990; Srkalovic et al. 1990). The heterogeneous distribution of somatostatin receptors in human breast biopsies has been reported, indicating that the size of the analyzed biopsies could influence the percentage of positive tumors (Reubi et al. 1990). Using ^{111}In-octreotide scintigraphy (Krenning et al. 1991) and ^{125}I-BIM-23014C cross-linking assay, 78% and 90% of breast tumors were considered positive for somatostatin receptors, respectively (Prévost et al. 1992).

Contradictory correlations between somatostatin receptor and sex-steroid receptors have been described. Reubi and Torhorst (1989) found a positive correlation between somatostatin receptors and steroid receptors in 36 tumors, but no correlation with these parameters was found by us (Prévost et al. 1992). A highly significant correlation was established between the expression of neuroendocrine markers (chromogranin A, chromogranin B, synaptophysin) and high somatostatin receptor density in a series of 100 cases (Papotti et al. 1989). These findings are additional evidence of the existence of a group of breast cancers which have morphological and cytochemical similarities with neuroendocrine tumors.

The molecular heterogeneity of the somatostatin receptor, suggested by its ligand- and tissue-selective binding (Murthy et al. 1990) and marked variations in binding affinities for several somatostatin analogues (Srkalovic et al. 1990), was also demonstrated in breast cells. Distinct proteins complexed with somatostatin and the somatostatin analogue ^{125}I-BIM-23014C were revealed in human breast cancer cells using the cross-linking assay (Prévost et al. 1992). One BIM-23014C-specific complex (57 kDa) was observed in MCF-7 (monolayer, nodule, and tumor) and T47D, three complexes (27, 42, and 57 kDa) were detected in MDAMB-231, and no complex was visible in HBL-100, a cell line established with epithelial cells from the milk of a nursing mother with no evidence of a breast lesion. A total of 27 of 30 human breast tumors (90%) had at least one BIM-23014C receptor. The simultaneous presence of the three BIM-23014C receptors was positively correlated ($p<0.05$) to the low amount of sex-steroid receptors (<20 fmol/mg): they were present in 7 of 8 tumors that were estrogen and progesterone receptor-negative compared with in 4 of 14 tumors that were estrogen and progesterone receptor-positive. Another positive correlation was established between the absence of progesterone receptors and the presence of these three complexes, which were present in 12 of 16 progesterone receptor-negative versus 4 of 14 progesterone receptor-positive tumors. These three complexes were similar to those observed in pituitary cells using the same cross-linking assay (Murthy et al. 1990). The molecular weight of one of these complexes (42 kDa) is compatible with the two pancreatic somatostatin receptors (SST-R) SST-R1 and SST-R2 cloned by Yamada et al. (1992).

Apart from the therapeutic use of SST-R, the presence of SST-R may have prognostic significance, and additionally determining the receptor status for EGF, IGF-I, GH, PRL, somatostatin, estrogen, and progesterone in human breast cancer may lead to a more rational endocrine therapy. The prognostic significance of somatostatin receptors in breast cancer was mainly evaluated in one study (Foekens et al. 1989, 1990). The relapse-free survival for patients with tumors containing SST-R was significantly longer than for patients with SST-R-negative tumors (82% versus 46% disease free after 5 years; $p=0.04$). SST-R assays were performed by incubating a cryostat section with ^{125}I-SMS-204-090. The low amount of somatostatin receptor-positive tumors (15%) must be noted. Further studies are currently being performed to confirm this prognostic value.

Somatostatin Immunoreactivities in Breast Cells

The presence of immunoreactive somatostatin has been investigated by immunohistochemistry in 40 biopsies from breast cancer patients (Ciocca et al. 1990). Immunoreactivity was absent in normal mammary tissue and present in about 30% of the tumoral samples. This presence was also detected in culture. Human breast cell lines (ZR-75, MDAMB-436 and MCF-7) were found to synthesize somatostatin detected by immunoreactivity assay in the culture media (Nelson et al. 1989). The secretion of somatostatin by these cells suggests a possible autocrine or/and paracrine role for this peptide in the development of breast tumors.

Clinical Data

As already mentioned, the clinical data are still very scarce, mainly because it is difficult to get stable long-acting derivatives that can be of clinical use. In a phase II study with BIM-23014C, we elected to treat breast cancer patients with progressing metastatic disease and who were unresponsive to any other therapy, including hormonal manipulations (Morère et al. 1989). No data were obtained about the presence of somatostatin receptors. Of 30 patients reported and evaluable who had metastatic deposits in the liver and the lung and were thus not subjected to biopsies, a minor response was registered in 2, and in 13 the disease stabilized for a mean duration of 4 months although it had previously been progressing. Gastrointestinal toxicity was mild and transient. We are waiting for stable derivatives in order to resume clinical studies.

Regarding the future clinical use of somatostatin and somatostatin analogues, it seems possible to express the following considerations and guidelines:

1. Various somatostatin receptors should be measured in tissue samples prior to therapy. It is not yet known whether they are equally present in the primary tumor and its metastases.
2. An a posteriori correlation should be made with the presence of estrogen receptors because of the controversial findings mentioned above. It is not known if hormone receptors are required for an antimitogenic effect of somatostatin to be observed, even in the presence of somatostatin receptors.
3. Somatostatin in vitro induces apoptosis, which is not surprising since it opposes several growth factors, especially IGF-I. It ensures that a more differentiated stage is probably induced first. This probable differentiating effect could by itself modify the phenotype and perhaps lead to hormone receptor expression. In addition, somatostatin could be synergistic with other differentiating agents such as retinoic acid, 1–25 dihydroxy-vitamin D, suramin, and interferon-α (Klijn et al. 1990; Manni et al. 1989). These points can only be clarified through randomized controlled clinical trials.

Conclusion

The inhibitory activity of the somatostatin analogues demonstrated both in vivo and in vitro, the high percentage of somatostatin receptor-positive biopsies, and the absence of in vivo toxic effects are all factors that would support the clinical potential of somatostatin analogues in the treatment of breast cancer.

Moreover, the characterization of different subtypes of somatostatin receptors must lead to the development of new analogues (Murphy et al. 1990). These new molecules will be developed to have an enhanced direct inhibitory activity on cell proliferation and an enhanced inhibitory effect on the secretion of pituitary cells.

The prognostic value of somatostatin receptors is still unclear with regard to the high variation in the percentage of somatostatin receptor-positive biopsies. Determination of the subtype that is implicated in the definition of this prognostic parameter could clarify the significance of its value. The roles of somatostatin receptors in biopsies and of breast-secreted somatostatin remain unclear during the development of normal and tumoral breast. More information could pinpoint the exact physiological importance of this peptide/receptor pair and increase the efficiency of treatment with different somatostatin analogues.

References

Bogden AE, Taylor JE, Moreau JP, Coy DH (1990) Treatment of R-3327 prostate tumors with a somatostatin analogue (somatuline) as adjuvant therapy following surgical castration. Cancer Res 50:2646–2650

Brazeau P, Vale W, Burgas R, Ling N, Butscher M, Rivier J, Guillemin R (1973) Hypothalamic polypeptides that inhibit the secretion of immunoreactive pituitary growth hormone. Science 179:77–79

Ciocca DR, Puy LA, Fasoli LC Tello O, Aznar JC, Gago FE, Papa SI, Sonego R (1990) Corticotropin releasing hormone, luteinizing hormone releasing hormone, growth hormone releasing hormone and somatostatin like immunoreactivities in biopsies from breast cancer patients. Breast Cancer Res Treatment 15:175–184

Fekete M, Wittliff A, Schally AV (1989) Characteristics and distribution of receptors for (D-Trp^6)-Luteinizing-releasing hormone, somatostatin, epidermal growth factor, and sex steroids in 500 biopsy samples of human breast cancer. J Clin Lab Anal 3:137–147

Foekens JA, Portengen H, van Putten WLJ, Trapman AM, Reubi JC, Alexia-Figusch S, Klijn JGM (1989) Prognostic value of receptors for insulin-like growth factor, somatostatin, and epidermal growth factor in human breast cancer. Cancer Res 49:7002–7009

Foekens JA, van Putten W, Portengen H, Rodenburg CJ, Reubi JC, Berns PM, Henzen-Logmans SC, van der Burg M, Klijn JMG (1990) Prognostic value of pS2 protein and receptors for epidermal growth factor, insulin-like growth factor I and somatostatin in patients with breast and ovarian cancer. J Steroid Biochem Mol Biol 37:815–821

Ghirlanda G, Ucciolo L, Perri F, Almonte L, Bertoli A, Manna R, Frati L, Greco AV (1983) Epidermal growth factor, somatostatin and psoriasis. Lancet i(8):65

Kimura N, Hayafuji C, Konagaya H, Takahashi K (1986) 17 beta-estradiol induces somatostatin (SRIF) inhibition of prolactin release and regulates SRIF receptors in rat anterior pituitary cells. Endocrinology 119:1028–1036

Klijn JGM, Setyono-Han B, Bakker GH, van der Burg MEL et al. (1990) Growth factor receptor pathway interfering treatment by somatostatin analogs and suramin: preclinical and clinical studies. J Steroid Biochem Mol Biol 37:1089–1095

Krenning EP, Lamberts SWJ, Reubi JC, Kwekkeboom DJ (1991) 111-In octreotide in scintigraphy in oncology. Congress on Sandostatin, Monté-Carlo, p 39

Manni A, Boucher AE, Demers LM, Harvey HA, Lipton A, Simmonds MA, Bartholomew M (1989) Endocrine effects of combined somatostatin analog and bromocriptine therapy in women with advanced breast cancer. Breast Cancer Res Treat 14:289–298

McGuire WL, Dickson RB, Osborne CK, Salomon D (1988) The role of growth factors in breast cancer. Breast Cancer Res Treat 12:159–166

Morère JF, Cour V, Breau JL, Boaziz C, Basin C, Israël L (1989) Stabilizing effect of BIM23014, a long acting somatostatin analog in 30 cases of advanced breast cancer: a phase II study. Proc Am Soc Clin Oncol 8: abstract 179

Murphy WA, Taylor JE, Moreau S, Moreau JP (1990) New octapeptide analogs of somatostatin with enhanced in vitro activity and receptor affinity. 72nd annual meeting of the American endocrine society, Atlanta, GA, June 20–23, 1990, abstract 518, p. 154

Murthy KK, Srikant CB, Patel Y (1990) Evidence for multiple protein constituents of the somatostatin receptor in pituitary tumor cells: affinity cross-linking and molecular characterization. Endocrinology 125:948–956

Nelson J, Cremin M, Murphy RF (1989) Synthesis of somatostatin by breast cancer cells and their inhibition by exogenous somatostatin and sandostatin. Br J Cancer 59:739–742

Pagliacci MC, Tognellini R, Grignani F, Nicoletti I (1991) Inhibition of human breast cancer cell (Mcf7) growth in vitro by the somatostatin analog SMS201-995 effects on cell cycle parameters and apoptotic cell death. Endocrinology 129:255–256

Papotti M, Macri L, Bussolati G, Rebi JC (1989) Correlative study on neuroendocrine differentiation and presence of somatostatin receptors in breast carcinomas. Int J Cancer 43:365–369

Prévost G, Gonzalez W, Thomas F (1991 a) La somatostatine et ses analogues dans le traitement du cancer du sein. Cah Cancerol 3:3–10

Prévost G, Foehrlé E, Thomas F, Pihan I, Veber N, Starzec A, Israel L (1991 b) Growth of human breast cancer cells inhibited by the somatostatin analogue BIM23014 (somatuline). Endocrinology 128:323–330

Prévost G, Lanson M, Thomas F, Veber N, Gonzalez W, Beaupain R, Starzec A, Bogden A (1992) Molecular heterogeneity of somatostatin analogue BIM23014C receptors in human breast carcinoma using cross-linking assay. Cancer Res 52:843–850

Reubi JC, Torhorst J (1989) The relationship between somatostatin, epidermal growth factor, and steroid hormone receptors in breast cancer. Cancer 64:1254–1260

Reubi JC, Maurer R, von Keder K, Torhost J, Klijn JGM, Lamberts SWJ (1987) Somatostatin receptors in human endocrine tumors. Cancer Res 47:551–558

Reubi JC, Waser B, Foekens JA, Klijn JG, Lamberts SWJ, Laissue J (1990) Somatostatin receptor incidence and distribution in breast cancer using receptor autoradiography: relationship to EGF receptor. Int J Cancer 46:416–420

Scambia G, Benedetti Panici P, Baiocchi P, Perrone L, Iacobelli S, Mancuso S (1988) Antiproliferative effects of somatostatin and the somatostatin analog SMS201-995 on three human breast cancer cell lines. J Cancer Res Clin Oncol 114:306–308

Setyono-Han B, Henkelman MS, Foekens JA, Klijn JGM (1987) Direct inhibitory effects of somatostatin (analogues) on the growth of human breast cancer cells. Cancer Res 47:1566–1570

Stolfi R, Parisi AM, Natoli C, Iacobelli S (1990) Advanced breast cancer: response to somatostatin. Anticancer Res 10:203–204

Srkalovic G, Cai R, Schally A (1990) Evaluation of receptors for somatin in various tumors using different analogs. Endocrinology 70:661–669

Szende B, Lapis K, Redding W, Srkalovic G, Schally A (1989) Growth inhibition of MTX mammary carcinoma by enhancing programmed cell death (apoptosis) with LH-RH and somatostatin. Breast Cancer Res Treat 14:307–314

Taylor J, Bogden A, Moreau JP, Coy D (1988) In vitro and in vivo inhibition of human small cell lung carcinoma (NCI-H69) growth by a somatostatin analogue. Biochem Biophys Res Commun 153:81–86

Thomas F, Parmar A, Prévost G, Kuhn JM, Moreau JP, Bogden A (1991) Les analogues de la somatostatine en cancérologie. Bull Cancer 78:693–707

Thomas F, Bogden A, Moreau JP (1992) Somatuline, a somatostatin analogue inhibits the growth of human and rat breast cancer cell lines in vivo. In: Fibeg HH, Berger DP (eds) Immunodeficient mice in oncology. Karger, Basel (Contributions to Oncology, Vol 42) (in press)

Vennin P, Peyrat JP, Bonneterre J, Louchez MM, Harris AG, Demaille A (1989) Effect of the long-acting somatostatin analogue SMS201-995 (sandostatin) in advanced breast cancer. Anticancer Res 9:153–156

Weber C, Merriam L, Koschitzky T, Karp F, Benson M, Logerfo P (1989) Inhibition of growth of human breast carcinomas in vivo by somatostatin analog SMS201-995: treatment of nude mouse xenografts. Surgery 106:416–422

Weckbecker G, Bruns C, Liu R, Tolscsvai L, Pless J (1990) Growth inhibitory effect of SMS201-995 in cell and animal cancer models. Growth factors and their receptors in cancer, Congress of Houston, p 112 (abstract 61)

Yamada Y, Post SR, Wang K, Tager HS, Bell GI, Seino S (1992) Cloning and functional characterization of a family of human and mouse somatostatin receptors expressed in brain gastrointestinal tract and kidney. Proc Natl Acad Sci 89:251–255

Yee D, Paik S, Lebovic GS, Marcus RR, Favoni RE, Cullen KJ, Lippman ME, Rosen N (1989) Analysis of insulin-like growth factor I gene expression in malignancy: evidence for a paracrine role in human breast cancer. Mol Endocrinol 3:509–517

Somatostatin Analogues and Small-Cell Lung Carcinoma

J. E. Taylor

Biomeasure Inc., 9–15 Avenue E, Hopkinton, MA 01748, USA

Introduction

Small-cell lung carcinoma (SCLC), which comprises approximately 25% of all new cases of lung cancer, is characterized by the expression of distinct neuroendocrine markers. These include cytoplasmic secretory granules, L-Dopa decarboxylase, neuron-specific enolase, and creatine kinase-BB (Carney et al. 1985; Carney 1991, 1992). Another significant property initially observed for SCLC is the presence of autocrine peptide or polypeptide growth factor loops for the gastrin-releasing peptide (GRP)/bombesin/neuromedin B family of peptides (Moody et al. 1983; Cuttitta et al. 1985; Cardona et al. 1991; Corjay et al. 1991), transferrin (Vostrejs et al. 1988), and insulin-like growth factor I (Nakanishi et al. 1988). Subsequent studies have additionally shown that multiple peptides and their respective receptors, e.g., bradykinin, neurotensin, cholecystokinin, substance P, vasoactive intestinal peptide, vasopressin, calcitonin, adrenocorticotrophic hormone (ACTH), can be detected in various SCLC cell lines (Bepler et al. 1988; Viallet and Minna 1989; Carney 1991, 1992; Woll 1991 a, b), and these peptides may also function as autocrine or paracrine factors (Sethi et al. 1992). In addition to growth-promoting factors, tachykinin (Bepler et al. 1987, 1988), opioid (Roth and Barchas 1986; Maneckjee and Minna 1990), and somatostatin (somatotropin release inhibiting factor, SRIF) peptides may operate as autocrine growth-inhibitory factors for SCLC (Sorenson et al. 1981; Taylor et al. 1988 a, b). These observations indicate that SCLC growth may be regulated in a complex manner by a combination of several positive (mitogenic) and negative (antimitogenic) autocrine loops, and that disruption of the mitogenic influence or enhancement of the antimitogenic loop could lead to a diminution of tumor growth. With respect to SRIF peptides, it is highly interesting that SCLC is derived from the bronchial epithelium, which is not normally considered a physiologically responsive tissue to SRIF. Consequently, this led to the possibility that SRIF peptides could be exploited pharmacologically to selectively target SCLC as antiproliferative peptides. The investigations of this proposition have focused on the

Recent Results in Cancer Research, Vol. 129

following lines of research and are reviewed in this chapter: (a) in vitro SRIF receptor studies with SCLC tumor cell lines and solid tumors; (b) the effects on in vitro proliferation; and (c) the effects on in vivo/xenograft tumor models. The pharmacological growth experiments have employed the use of potent and metabolically stable SRIF octapeptide analogues (see Table 1), some of which are in clinical use or currently undergoing clinical trials for SCLC, as well as for the diagnosis and treatment of endocrine and several other types of malignancies. These other oncological applications of SRIF peptides are reviewed in other chapters in this volume and in previous reviews (Lamberts et al. 1987, 1990b, 1991; Schally 1988; Parmer et al. 1989; Lamberts 1988).

Table 1. [^{125}I-Tyr^{11}]SRIF-14 binding of human SCLC membranes

SCLC Cell line/tumor	Receptor concentration (fmol/mg protein)
NCI-H69	173 ± 2
NCI-H345	98 ± 22
NCI-H209	15 ± 4
NCI-N417	Not detectable
LX-1	Not detectable

SRIF Receptor Studies

High-affinity, saturable binding of radiolabeled SRIF to cultured SCLC cells was first described by Taylor et al. (1988a). This initial report which dealt with the in vitro binding of [^{125}I-Tyr^{11}]SRIF-14 to membranes prepared from the classical NCI-H69 SCLC cell line was fortuitous, as high receptor levels enabled a detailed characterization of the receptor pharmacology. In routine experiments, specific binding accounted for approximately 70% of the total radioligand bound at 0.05 nM, and saturation analysis of [^{125}I-Tyr^{11}]SRIF-14 binding yielded a K_d of 0.59 ± 0.02 nM and a receptor concentration of 173 ± 2 fmol/mg protein. Saturable binding ($B_{max} = 12.5$ fmol/mg protein) was also expressed in solid NCI-H69 tumors established by serial transplantation and grown in athymic nude mice. Other classical SCLC cell lines (NCI-H345, NCI-H209) were also enriched in SRIF receptors, albeit in lower concentrations (Table 1). Interestingly, the variant SCLC cell line NCI-N417 and the poorly differentiated solid SCLC tumor LX-1 did not exhibit detectable [^{125}I-Tyr^{11}]SRIF-14 binding, but responded to the antiproliferative actions of SRIF octapeptide analogues (Bogden et al. 1990b). Employing in vitro receptor autoradiographic techniques, Macaulay et al. (1991) also observed SRIF receptors in three of four established SCLC lines, but not in two non-small-cell lines. In addition to established in vitro SCLC cell lines, SRIF receptors have been detected autoradiographically in two of four primary tumor samples (Reubi et al. 1990a), and in a similar study, two of three biopsy samples were receptor positive (Sagman et al. 1990). Of these combined studies, none of 17 non-small-cell lung carcinoma samples had SRIF receptors. SCLC tumors have also been detected visually in humans after the injection of [^{123}I]Tyr^3-octreotide (Lamberts et al. 1990a; Kwekkeboom et al. 1991) or [^{111}I-DTPA]D-Phe^1-octreotide (Krenning et al. 1992).

Pharmacological specificity studies have demonstrated that both SRIF-28 and SRIF-14, as well as antiproliferative SRIF octapeptide analogues, were potent inhibitors (approximately 0.3–3 n*M* IC_{50}) of [^{125}I-Tyr^{11}]SRIF-14 binding to SCLC NCI-H69 membranes (Table 2). Hill slopes were in the range of 0.85–1.2 for all peptides, indicating the presence of a single class of receptor sites. Example inhibition curves are shown in Fig. 1. The relationship of the SCLC SRIF receptor to the recently cloned receptor subtypes (Yamada et al. 1992; Kluxen et al. 1992) or other putative subtypes reported in the literature are unknown (Reubi 1984; Tran et al. 1985; Raynor and Reisine 1989; Martin et al. 1991). However, the observation that the synthetic SRIF octapeptide analogues BIM-23014 and SMS201-995 bind with high affinity to an apparent single site on the NCI-H69 membranes seems to indicate that the SCLC receptor is more similar to the peripheral SRIF receptor than that observed in the brain (Heiman et al. 1987). Numerous studies have also shown that SRIF receptors in various tissues can be coupled to G proteins, as shown by the effects of GTP or GTP analogues on SRIF receptor binding and pertussis toxin sensitivity to SRIF biological activity (Hsu et al. 1991; Law et al. 1991; Murray-Whelan and Schlegel 1992; Pan et al. 1992; Rens-Domiano and Reisine 1992). Receptor-specific [^{125}I-Tyr^{11}]SRIF-14 binding to SCLC NCI-H69 membranes is inhibited by the nonhydrolyzable GTP analogue Gpp(NH)p (Fig. 2), suggesting that the inhibition of SCLC proliferation by SRIF peptides may be mediated through G protein membrane/transduction

Table 2. In vitro inhibition of [^{125}I-Tyr^{11}]SRIF-14 binding to human SCLC NCI-H69 membranes

SRIF peptide	IC_{50} (n*M*)
SRIF-28 Ser-Ala-Asn-Ser-Asn-Pro-Ala-Met-Ala-Pro-Arg-Glu-Arg-Lys-Ala-Gly cyclo[Cys-Lys-Asn-Phe-Phe-Trp-Lys-Thr-Phe-Thr-Ser-Cys]-OH	0.49 ± 0.12
SRIF-14 Ala-Gly-cyclo[Cys-Lys-Asn-Phe-Phe-Trp-Lys-Thr-Phe-Thr-Ser-Cys]-OH	3.2 ± 0.8
BIM-23014 (somatuline) 3-(2-naphthyl)-D-Ala-cyclo[Cys-Try-D-Trp-Lys-Val-Cys]-Thr-NH_2	0.66 ± 0.25
BIM-23034 D-Phe-cyclo[Cys-Tyr-D-Trp-Lys-Val-Cys]-3-(2-naphthyl)-D-Ala-NH_2	2.1 ± 0.6
SMS 201-995 (sandostatin, octreotide) D-Phe-cyclo[Cys-Phe-D-Trp-Lys-Thr-Cys-]Thr(ol)	0.49 ± 0.14
RC-160 D-Phe-cyclo[Cys-Tyr-D-Trp-Lys-Val-Cys]Trp-NH_2	0.28 ± 0.01

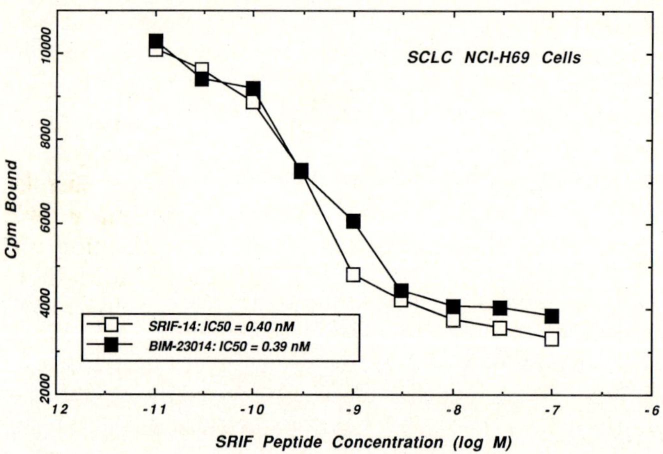

Fig. 1. In vitro inhibition of [^{125}I-Tyr^{11}]SRIF-14 binding to cultured human SCLC NCI-H69 membranes

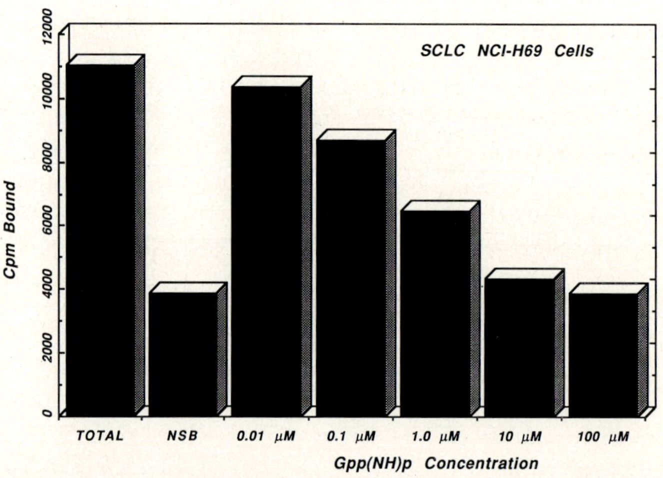

Fig. 2. In vitro inhibition of [^{125}I-Tyr^{11}]SRIF-14 binding to cultured human SCLC NCl-H69 membranes by Gpp(NH)p

mechanisms. Several laboratories have reported that the antiproliferative action of SRIF peptides may be related to the stimulation of phosphotyrosine phosphatase activity (Liebow et al. 1989, 1990; Cambillau et al. 1990; Lee et al. 1991), possibly through a G protein coupled mechanism (Pan et al. 1992). The phosphatase hypothesis was developed, however, using epidermal growth factor (EGF) receptor-positive tumors, and may not be relevant to SCLC tumors which lack EGF receptors (Reubi et al. 1990b; Moody et al. 1990).

In Vitro Growth Inhibition Studies

Several reports have demonstrated that established in vitro SCLC cell lines are sensitive to the antiproliferative activity of SRIF peptides. In vitro growth-inhibitory activity was first reported for the potent and endocrinologically active SRIF analogue BIM-23014 (Heiman et al. 1987; Taylor et al. 1988 a; Sassolas et al. 1989; Moreau et al. 1991), against the NCI-H69 SCLC cell line growth in liquid culture (Taylor et al. 1988 b). In this case, cell proliferation was significantly decreased by incubation with low concentrations of BIM-23014 (Fig. 3, bottom panel). BIM-23014 and BIM-23034 were also active as antiproliferative peptides in clonogenic assays of SCLC cell proliferation (Fig. 3, top panel; Taylor et al. 1991). The potency range (0.1 – 1000 nM) was similar to that observed for the inhibition of [^{125}I-Tyr^{11}]SRIF-14 binding to SCLC NCI-H345 membranes. Utilizing [^{3}H]thymidine incorporation as a measure of in vitro cell growth, Macaulay et al. (1991) reported that only one of three SRIF receptor-positive, established SCLC cell lines responded to SMS201-995 (octreotide). In spite of the apparent discrepancies between receptor status and in vitro growth inhibition, these data indicate that SRIF analogues can have a direct antiproliferative action. This direct activity may result from the disruption of autocrine growth cycles through the inhibition of growth factor release (Kee et al. 1988; Taylor et al. 1991).

In Vivo Growth Inhibition Studies

The initial demonstration of in vivo inhibitory activity of SCLC by an SRIF analogue was made by Taylor et al. (1988 b), who reported that the appearance of measurable tumors and growth of NCI-H69 cells implanted subcutaneously into athymic nude mice (first transplant generation) was effectively slowed by intraperitoneal injections (500 μg/mouse). Subcutaneous infusion around the tumor resulted in the development of only small palpable tumors which regressed in size. There was an obvious acceleration of tumor growth in both the intraperitoneal and subcutaneous infusion groups following termination of peptide treatment, indicating that the tumor-inhibitory effects were antiproliferative rather than cytotoxic. BIM-23014 was also active against in vivo propagated SCLC NCI-H69 tumors derived from a solid tumor donor (second transplant generation).

Our laboratory has examined the effects of BIM-23014 on the growth of other SCLC implanted subcutaneously as tumor xenografts in athymic nude mice (Bodgen et al. 1990 b). BIM-23014 retarded the growth of NCI-N417, NCI-H345, and the LX-1 SCLC tumors. Figure 4 summarizes these results along with those for the NCI-H69 second transplant generation tumor. BIM-23014 was most effective when administered as a perilesional subcutaneous infusion, and, again, withdrawal of SRIF peptide treatment resulted in tumor regrowth. In addition, we have also observed marked growth-inhibitory effects with the SRIF octapeptide analogue BIM-23034 (Fig. 5), previously shown to

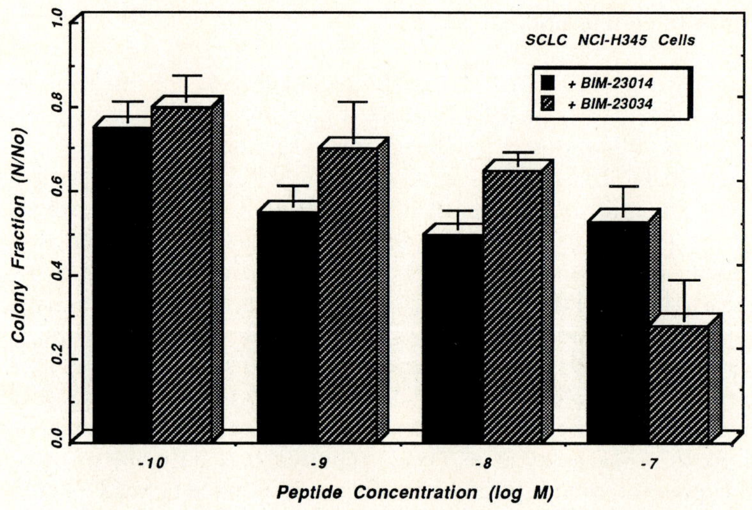

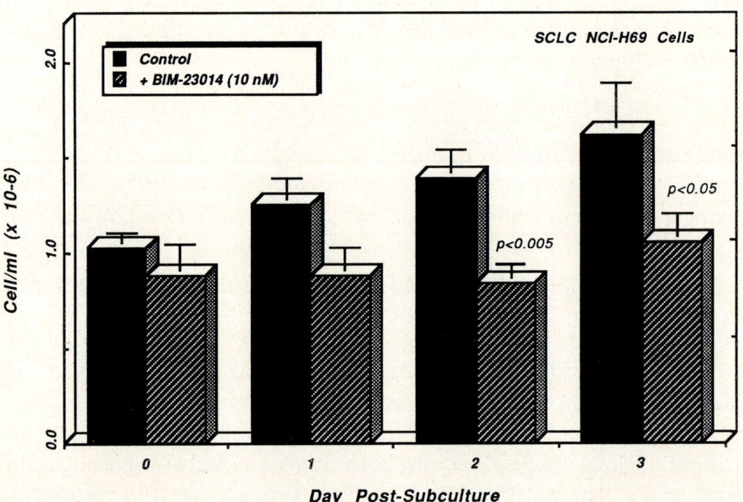

Fig. 3. *Top panel*, in vitro inhibition of clonal human SCLC NCI-H345 growth by the SRIF octapeptide analogues, BIM-23014 (3-(2-naphthyl-D-Ala-cyclo[Cys-Try-D-Trp-Lys-Val-Cys]-Thr-NH_2) and BIM-23034 (D-Phe-cyclo[Cys-Tyr-D-Trp-Lys-Val-Cys]-3-(2-naphthyl)-D-Ala-NH_2). *Bottom panel*, in vitro inhibition of human SCLC NCI-H69 cell proliferation in liquid culture by the SRIF octapeptide analogue, BIM-23014 (D-Phe-cyclo[Cys-Tyr-D-Trp-Lys-Val-Cys]-3-(2-naphthyl)-D-Ala-NH_2)

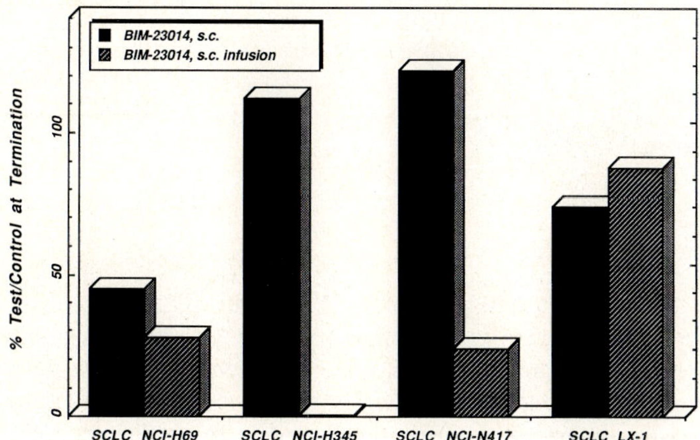

Fig. 4. Response (percent age test/control at termination) of human SCLC NCI-H69 (second transplant generation solid tumor), NCI-H345 (transplanted from in vitro cell culture), NCI-N417 (transplanted from in vitro cell culture), and LX-1 (established solid tumor maintained by serial transplantation) xenografts to BIM-23014 (3-(2-naphthyl)-D-Ala-cyclo[Cys-Try-D-Trp-Lys-Val-Cys]-Thr-NH_2) administered at 500 µg per injection (twice daily, every day) subcutaneously on the side opposite of tumor, or as a subcutaneous infusion around the tumor. The treatment durations were 40, 87, 49, and 26 days for the H69, H345, N417, and LX-1 tumors, respectively

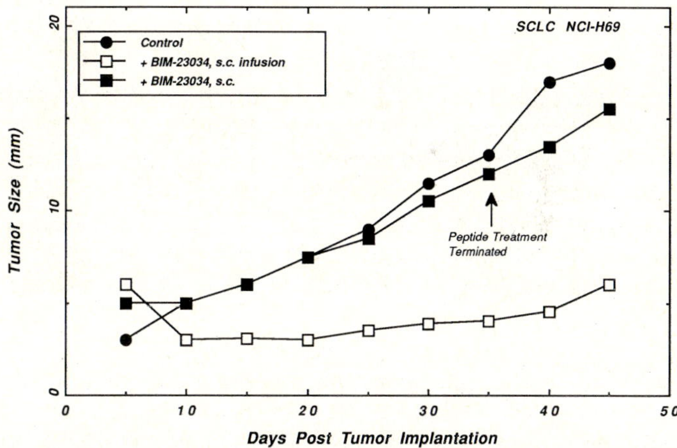

Fig. 5. Response (tumor size in millimeters) of human SCLC NHI-H69 xenografts to the SRIF octapeptide (D-Phe-cyclo[Cys-Tyr-D-Trp-Lys-Val-Cys]-3-(2-naphthyl)-D-Ala-NH_2) administered at 250 µg per injection (twice daily, every day) subcutaneously on the side opposite of tumor, or as subcutaneous infusion around the tumor. Tumors were measured two or three times weekly with Vernier calipers, and tumor size was calculated as the average of two diameters (length + width)/2 mm

be active in vitro (Taylor et al. 1991). For all in vivo studies, perilesional infusion was clearly superior to subcutaneous or intraperitoneal administration, which emphasizes the importance of the peptide reaching the tumor in concentrations which are sufficient to antagonize the actions of endogenous growth-promoting factors.

Conclusions

The primary endogenous SRIF peptide SRIF-14 (Ala-Gly-cyclo[Cys-Lys-Asn-Phe-Phe-Trp-Lys-Thr-Phe-Thr-Ser-Cys]-OH) was originally isolated from the hypothalamus and characterized by its property to inhibit the anterior pituitary secretion of growth hormone (Reichlin 1983a, b). SRIF and SRIF receptors are also widely distributed in the brain and peripheral tissues and function in the regulation of endocrine and exocrine pancreatic function. SRIF is inhibitory to gastrointestinal blood flow and secretory activity and may also be a neurotransmitter or neuromodulator in the brain (Epelbaum 1986; Gulya et al. 1985; Moyse et al. 1989; Vécsei and Widerlöv 1990; Martin et al. 1991; Raynor and Reisine 1992). In view of these physiological actions of SRIF, it was not surprising that SRIF or SRIF analogues were initially employed experimentally and clinically to either inhibit the growth or retard the secretory activity of endocrine or exocrine tumors, i.e., pancreatic carcinoma and acromegaly, derived from tissues that are normally responsive to the biological actions of SRIF (DeFeudis and Moreau 1986; Moreau and DeFeudis 1987; Reubi et al. 1987; Lamberts 1988; Parmer et al. 1989; Lamberts et al. 1990b, 1991; Vance and Harris 1991).

Interestingly, SRIF receptors were reported to be expressed in SCLC, a malignancy derived from a tissue not normally considered as a biological target of SRIF, and the observed in vitro action demonstrated that SRIF peptides had an antiproliferative activity which was independent of its effects on pituitary GH secretion and possibly related to an interruption of dysregulated autocrine or paracrine/peptide growth systems.

Additional studies with the SRIF analogue BIM-23014 against other nonendocrine tumors have also demonstrated SRIF receptors and either in vitro or/and in vivo activity against breast carcinomas, hepatomas, prostate melanoma, and neuroblastoma (DeFeudis and Moreau 1986; Moreau and DeFeudis 1987; Murphy et al. 1987; Bogden et al. 1988, 1990a), and the other structurally related octapeptide SRIF analogues SMS201-995 and RC-160 have also been shown to be active as inhibitors of breast (Setyono-Han et al. 1987; Nelson et al. 1989; Papotti et al. 1989; Weber et al. 1989; Stolfi et al. 1990) and prostate tumor (Schally and Redding 1987; Siegel et al. 1988) growth. These observations clearly indicate that (a) SRIF may have a generalized physiological role as a growth factor antagonist and may be involved in the 'fine tuning' of both endocrine and nonendocrine tumor growth or proliferation by acting as a negative modulator of local proliferation factors; and (b) the pharmacological magnification of this antiproliferative activity with potent and stable SRIF analogues can result in effective retardation of SCLC growth in experimental models, as well as for other and nonendocrine neoplasms. Clinical studies are currently in progress to evaluate this hypothesis in human SCLC patients.

References

Bepler G, Carney DN, Gazdar AF, Minna JD (1987) In vitro growth inhibition of human small cell lung cancer by physalaemin. Cancer Res 47:2371–2375

Bepler G, Rotsch M, Jaques G, Haeder M, Heymanns J, Hartogh G, Kiefer P, Havemann K (1988) Peptides and growth factors in small cell lung cancer: production, binding sites, and growth effects. J Cancer Res Clin Oncol 114:235–244

Bogden AE, Taylor JE, Moreau J-P, Coy DH, Moreau S, LePage DJ (1988) In vivo responsiveness of human and animal tumors to Somatostatin (SRIF) analogue BIM-23014C (DC13-116). Proc AARC 29:56

Bogden AE, Taylor JE, Moreau J-P, Coy DH (1990a) Treatment of R-3327 prostate tumors with a somatostatin analogue (Somatuline) as adjuvant therapy following surgical castration. Cancer Res 50:2646–2650

Bogden AE, Taylor JE, Moreau J-P, Coy DH, Le Page DJ (1990b) Response of human lung tumor xenografts to treatment with a somatostatin analogue (Somatuline). Cancer Res 50:4360–4365

Cambillau C, Tahiri-Jouti N, Bascail L, Viguerie N, Vidal C, Vaysse N, Susini C (1990) Antiproliferative effect of somatostatin: possible involvement of a membrane phosphotyrosine phosphatase. Digestion 46 [Suppl I]:38 (Abstract)

Cardona C, Rabbitts PH, Spindel ER, Ghatei MA, Bleehen NM, Bloom SR, Reeve JG (1991) Production of neuromedin B and neuromedin B gene expression in human lung tumor cell lines. Cancer Res 51:5205–5211

Carney DN (1991) Lung cancer biology. Eur J Cancer 27:366–369

Carney DN (1992) Biology of small-cell lung cancer. Lancet 339:843–846

Carney DN, Gazdar AF, Bepler G, Guccion JG, Marangos PJ, Moody TW, Zweig MH, Minna JD (1985) Establishment and identification of small cell lung cancer cell lines having classic and variant features. Cancer Res 45:2913–2923

Corjay MH, Dobrzanski DJ, Way JM, Viallet J, Shapira H, Worland P, Sausville EA, Battey JM (1991) Two distinct bombesin receptor subtypes are expressed and functional in human lung carcinoma cells. J Biol Chem 266:18771–18779

Cuttitta F, Carney DN, Mulshine J, Moody TW, Fedorko J, Fischler A, Minna JD (1985) Bombesin-like peptides can function as autocrine growth factors in human small-cell lung cancer. Nature 316:823–826

DeFeudis FV, Moreau J-P (1986) Studies on somatostatin analogues might lead to new therapies for certain types of cancer. TiPS 7:384–386

Epelbaum J (1986) Somatostatin in the central nervous system: physiology and pathological modifications. Prog Neurobiol 27:63–100

Gulya K, Wamsley JK, Gehlert D, Pelton JT, Duckles SP, Hruby VJ, Yamamura HI (1985) Light microscopic autoradiographic localization of somatostatin receptors in the rat brain. J Pharmacol Exp Ther 235:254–258

Heiman ML, Murphy WA, Coy DH (1987) Differential binding of somatostatin agonists to somatostatin receptors in brain and adenohypophysis. Neuroendocrinol 45:429–436

Hsu WH, Xiang H, Rajan AS, Kunze DL, Boyd AE III (1991) Somatostatin inhibits insulin secretion by a G-protein-mediated decrease in Ca^{2+} entry through voltage-dependent Ca^{2+} channels in the beta cell. J Biol Chem 266:837–843

Kee KA, Finan TM, Korman LY, Moody TW (1988) Somatostatin inhibits the secretion of bombesin-like peptides from small cell lung cancer cells. Peptides 9 [Suppl I]:257–261

Kluxen F-W, Bruns C, Lubbert H (1992) Expression cloning of a rat brain somatostatin receptor cDNA. Proc Natl Acad Sci USA 89:4618–4622

Krenning EP, Bakker WH, Kooij PPM, Breeman WAP, Oei HY, de Jong OM, Reubi J-C, Visser TJ, Bruns C, Kwekkeboom DJ, Reijs AEM, van Hagen PM, Koper JW, Lamberts SWJ (1992) Somatostatin receptor scintigraphy with indium-111-DTPA-D-Phe-1-octreotide in man: metabolism, dosimetry and comparison with iodine-123-Tyr-3-octreotide. J Nucl Med 33:642–658

Kwekkeboom DJ, Krenning EP, Bakker WH, Oei HY, Splinter TAW, Kho GS, Lamberts SWJ (1991) Radioiodinated somatostatin analog scintigraphy in small-cell lung cancer. J Nucl Med 32:1845–1848

Lamberts SWJ (1988) The role of somatostatin in the regulation of anterior pituitary hormone secretion and the use of its analogs in the treatment of human pituitary tumors. Endocrine Rev 9:417–436

Lamberts SWJ, Koper JW, Reubi J-C (1987) Potential role of somatostatin analogues in the treatment of cancer. Eur J Clin Invest 17:281–287

Lamberts SWJ, Bakker WH, Reubi J-C, Krenning EP (1990a) Treatment with sandostatin and in vivo localization of tumors with radiolabeled somatostatin analogs. Metabolism 39:152–155

Lamberts SWJ, Krenning EP, Klijn JGM, Reubi J-C (1990b) Clinical applications of somatostatin analogs. Trends Endocrinol Metabol 1:139–144

Lamberts SWJ, Krenning EP, Reubi J-C (1991) The role of somatostatin and its analogs in the diagnosis and treatment of tumors. Endocrine Rev 12:450–482

Law SF, Manning D, Reisine T (1991) Identification of the subunits of GTP-binding proteins coupled to somatostatin receptors. J Biol Chem 266:17885–17897

Lee MT, Liebow C, Kamer AR, Schally AV (1991) Effects of epidermal growth factor and analogues of luteinizing hormone-releasing hormone and somatostatin on phosphorylation and dephosphorylation of tyrosine residues of specific protein substrates in various tumors. Proc Natl Acad Sci USA 88:1656–1660

Liebow C, Reilly C, Serrano M, Schally AV (1989) Somatostatin analogues inhibit growth of pancreatic cancer by stimulating tyrosine phosphatase. Proc Natl Acad Sci USA 86:2003–2007

Liebow C, Lee MT, Schally A (1990) Antitumor effects of somatostatin mediated by the stimulation of tyrosine phosphatase. Metabolism 39 [Suppl 2]:163–166

Macaulay VM, Smith IE, Everard MJ, Teale JD, Reubi J-C, Millar JL (1991) Experimental and clinical studies with somatostatin analogue octreotide in small cell lung cancer. Br J Cancer 64:451–456

Maneckjee R, Minna JD (1990) Opioid and nicotine receptors affect growth regulation on human lung cancer cell lines. Proc Natl Acad Sci USA 87:3294–3298

Martin J-L, Chesselet M-F, Raynor K, Gonzales C, Reisine T (1991) Differential distribution of somatostatin receptor subtypes in rat brain revealed by newly developed somatostatin analogs. Neuroscience 41:581–593

Moody TW, Bertness V, Carney DN (1983) Bombesin-like peptides and receptors in human tumor cell lines. Peptides 4:683–686

Moody TW, Lee M, Kris RM, Bellot F, Bepler G, Oie H, Gazdar AF (1990) Lung carcinoid cell lines have bombesin-like peptides and EGF receptors. J Cell Biochem 43:139–147

Moreau J-P, DeFeudis FV (1987) Pharmacological studies of somatostatin and somatostatin analogues: therapeutic advances and perspectives. Life Sci 40:419–437

Moreau S, Murphy WA, Coy DH (1991) Comparison of somatuline (BIM-23014) and somatostatin on endocrine and exocrine activities in the rat. Drug Dev Res 22:79–93

Moyse E, Slama A, Videau C, de Angela P, Kordon C, Epelbaum J (1989) Regional distribution of somatostatin receptor affinity states in rat brain: effects of divalent cations and GTP. Reg Peptides 26:225–234

Murphy WA, Lance VA, Moreau S, Moreau J-P, Coy DH (1987) Inhibitions of rat prostate tumor growth by an octapeptide analog of somatostatin. Life Sci 40:2515–2522

Murray-Whelan R, Schlegel W (1992) Brain somatostatin receptor-G protein interaction. $G\alpha$ C-terminal antibodies demonstrate coupling of the soluble receptor with $G_{i(1-3)}$ but not with G_0. J Biol Chem 267:2960–2965

Nakanishi Y, Mulshine JL, Kaspryzk PG, Natale RB, Maneckjee R, Avis I, Treston AM, Gazdar AF, Minna JD, Cuttitta F (1988) Insulin-like growth factor-I can mediate autocrine proliferation of human small cell lung cancer cell lines in vitro. J Clin Invest 82:331–339

Nelson J, Cremin M, Murphy RF (1989) Synthesis of somatostatin by breast cancer cells and their inhibition by exogenous somatostatin and sandostatin. Br J Cancer 59:739–742

Pan GP, Florio T, Stork PJS (1992) G protein activation of a hormone-stimulated phosphatase in human tumor cells. Science 256:1215–1217

Papotti M, Macri L, Bussolati G, Reubi J-C (1989) Correlative study of neuroendocrine differentiation and presence of somatostatin receptors in breast carcinomas. Int J Cancer 43:365–369

Parmer H, Bodgen A, Mollard M, de Rouge B, Phillips RH, Lightman SL (1989) Somatostatin and somatostatin analogues in oncology. Cancer Treat Rev 16:95–115

Raynor K, Reisine T (1989) Analogs of somatostatin selectively label distinct subtypes of somatostatin receptors in rat brain. J Pharmacol Exp Ther 251:510–517

Raynor K, Reisine T (1992) Differential coupling of somatostatin 1 receptors to adenylyl cyclase in the rat striatum vs the pituitary and other regions of the rat brain. J Pharmacol Exp Ther 260:841–848

Reichlin S (1983a) Somatostatin. N Engl J Med 309:1495–1501

Reichlin S (1983b) Somatostatin. N Engl J Med 309:1556–1563

Rens-Domiano S, Reisine T (1992) Biochemical and functional properties of somatostatin receptors. J Neurochem 58:1987–1996

Reubi J-C (1984) Evidence for two somatostatin-14 receptor types in rat brain cortex. Neurosci Letters 49:259–263

Reubi J-C, Maurer R, Von Werder K, Torhorst J, Klijn JGM, Lamberts SWJ (1987) Somatostatin receptors in human endocrine tumors. Cancer Res 47:551–558

Reubi J-C, Kvols L, Krenning E, Lamberts SWJ (1990a) Distribution of somatostatin receptors in normal and tumor tissue. Metabolism 39 [Suppl 2]:78–81

Reubi J-C, Waser B, Sheppard M, Macaulay VM (1990b) Somatostatin receptors are present in small cell but not in non-small cell primary lung carcinomas: relationship to EGF-receptors. Int J Cancer 45:269–274

Roth KA, Barchas JD (1986) Small cell carcinoma cell lines contain opioid peptides and receptors. Cancer 57:769–773

Sagman U, Mullilns J, Kovacs K, Kerbel R, Ginsberg R, Reubi J-C (1990) Identification of somatostatin receptors in human lung carcinomas. Cancer 66:2129–2133

Sassolas G, Khalfallah Y, Chayvialle JA, Cohen R, Merabet S, Casez JP, Calvet P, Cabrera P (1989) Effects of the somatostatin analog BIM 23014 on the secretion of growth hormone, thyrotopin, and digestive peptides in normal men. J Clin Endocrinol Metab 68:239–246

Schally AV, Redding TW (1987) Somatostatin analogs as adjuncts to agonists of luteinizing hormone-releasing hormone in the treatment of experimental prostate cancer. Proc Natl Acad Sci USA 84:7275–7279

Schally AV (1988) Oncological applications of somatostatin analogues. Cancer Res 48:6977–6985

Sethi T, Langdon S, Smyth J, Rozengurt E (1992) Growth of small cell lung cancer cells: stimulation by multiple neuropeptides and inhibition by broad spectrum antagonists in vitro and in vivo. Cancer Res [Suppl] 52:2737s–2742s

Setyono-Han B, Henkelman MS, Foekens JA, Klijn JGM (1987) Direct inhibitory effects of somatostatin (analogues) on the growth of human breast cancer cells. Cancer Res 47:1566–1570

Siegel RA, Tolcsvai L, Rudin M (1988) Partial inhibition of the growth of transplanted Dunning rat prostate tumors with the long-acting somatostatin analogue Sandostatin (SMS 201-995). Cancer Res 48:4651–4655

Stolfi R, Parisi AM, Natoli C, Iacobelli S (1990) Advanced breast cancer: Response to somatostatin. Anticancer Res 10:203–204

Sorenson GD, Pettengill OS, Brinck-Johnsen T, Cate CC, Maurer LH (1981) Hormone production by cultures of small-cell carcinoma of the lung. Cancer 47:1289–1296

Taylor JE, Coy DH, Moreau J-P (1988a) High affinity binding of [^{125}I-Tyr^{11}]somatostatin-14 to human small cell lung carcinoma (NCI-H69). Life Sci 43:421–427

Taylor JE, Bogden AE, Moreau J-P, Coy DH (1988b) In vitro and in vivo inhibitions of human small cell lung carcinoma (NCI-H69) growth by a somatostatin analogue. Biochem Biophys Res Comm 153:81–86

Taylor JE, Moreau J-P, Baptiste L, Moody TW (1991) Octapeptide analogues of somatostatin inhibit the clonal growth and vasoactive intestinal peptide-stimulated cyclic AMP formation in human and small cell lung cancer cells. Peptides 12:839–843

Tran VT, Beal MF, Martin JB (1985) Two types of somatostatin receptors differentiated by cyclic somatostatin analogs. Science 228:492–495

Vance ML, Harris AG (1991) Long-term treatment of 189 acromegalic patients with the somatostatin analog octreotide. Arch Intern Med 151:1573–1578

Vécsei L, Widerlöv E (1990) Preclinical and clinical studies with somatostatin related to the central nervous system. Prog Neuro-Psycho Biol Psychiat 14:473–502

Viallet J, Minna JD (1989) Gastrin-releasing peptide (GRP, mammalian bombesin) in the pathogenesis of lung cancer. Prog Growth Factor Res 1:89–97

Vostrejs M, Moran P, Seligman P (1988) Transferrin synthesis by small cell lung cancer cells acts as an autocrine regulator of cellular proliferation. J Clin Invest 82:331–339

Weber C, Merriam L, Koschitzky T, Karp F, Benson M, Forde K, LoGerfo P (1989) Inhibition of growth of human breast carcinomas in vivo by somatostatin analog SMS 201-995: treatment of nude mouse xenografts. Surgery 106:416–422

Woll PJ (1991a) Neuropeptide growth factors and cancer. Br J Cancer 63:469–475

Woll PJ (1991b) Growth factors and lung cancer. Thorax 46:924–929

Yamada Y, Post SR, Wang K, Tager HS, Bell GI, Seing S (1992) Cloning and functional characterization of a family of human and mouse somatostatin receptors expressed in brain, gastrointestinal tract, and kidney. Proc Natl Acad Sci USA 89:251–255

Somatostatin and Neoplastic Pain

M. Kloke

Innere Klinik und Poliklinik (Tumorforschung), Westdeutsches Tumorzentrum, Universitätsklinikum Essen, Hufelandstraße 55, W-4300 Essen 1, FRG

Introduction

More than a dozen neuropeptides have been identified within the subset of sensory neurons, and there is increasing evidence that some of these peptides act as transmitters mediating slow synaptic potentials at primary afferent synapses. About 50% of small-diameter sensory neurons have so far been shown to contain neuropeptides. Most of them are found in the dorsal root ganglion and the superficial cells of the dorsal horn of the spinal column (Jessell and Dodd 1986). All we know is that their actions can be dissociated from that of the fast transmitters (Wall and Woolf 1986). They may be responsible for the long-latency, long-duration changes of excitability which influence activity triggered by fast neurotransmitters and participate in the second phase response of nociception (Ohkubo et al. 1990).

One of these neuropeptides is somatostatin (SST), which is present in small-diameter cells of the dorsal root ganglia associated with C-fiber afferents and in extrinsic and intrinsic dorsal horn fibers and terminals, with especially high concentrations in lamina II (Polak and Bloom 1986). Its role in physiological nociception and pain transmission has been the object of many studies which ended with partially conflicting results. Nevertheless, SST has been used as an analgesic in intractable cancer and severe postoperative pain. Since SST is degraded within minutes in serum, whereas in cerebrospinal fluid it is stable over a long period of time – probably due to the very low activity of peptidase in this compartment (Unger et al. 1988) it was administered in the peridural, subarachnoidal, or intraventricular space.

Results in Bioassays

Gaumann and Yaksh (1990) evaluated the effect of intrathecal SST on nociception and autonomic and motor function in rats. Whereas the occurrence of motor dysfunction was dose dependent, the blockade of nociception was ob-

Recent Results in Cancer Research, Vol. 129

served to varying degrees. Histological examination revealed mild or severe nucleolysis of the ventral and dorsal horns, giving clear evidence that SST was highly toxic, with no safety margin between antinociception and motor dysfunction. Similar neurotoxic effects characterized by truncal ataxia, dysmetria, and severe bradykinesia were observed by Leblanc et al. (1988) when they injected SST intracranially into primates; their response to pain was also reduced. Dirksen et al. (1990) demonstrated that the neurotoxic side effects of intrathecal SST in rats were related in incidence and degree to dose and interval, the antinociceptive potency being highest at short intervals. Kuraishi et al. (1985) and Tiseo et al. (1990) found that noxious thermal stimuli specifically increase the release of SST from the dorsal horn. And vice versa, SST induced inhibition of responses to noxious thermal but not mechanical stimulation. This suppression could not be antagonized by the μ-opiate antagonist naloxone (Sandkühler et al. 1990).

Therapeutic Use of SST as an Analgesic

Despite the disappointing results in animals, SST has been used as an analgesic in patients with acute and chronic pain. In 1984, Chrubasik first reported on eight patients who received intraventricular, intrathecal, or epidural SST, either for terminal cancer or postoperative pain over a period of maximum 8 days at a dosage of 10–125 µg/h (Chrubasik et al. 1984). They all obtained good pain relief which could not be antagonized by opiate antagonists. Two terminally ill patients received SST intrathecally for 60 days at rates up to 50 µg/h; adequate pain palliation was achieved and no toxicity mentioned (Meynadier et al. 1985). Epidural SST was not associated with any side effects, particularly any sedative effect, when administered to alleviate postoperative pain in eight patients at various dosages. Again the analgesic effect was not antagonized by naloxone (Chrubasik et al. 1985). It cannot be ruled out that four of these patients had been described in a former publication by Chrubasik et al. (1984). After intraventricular administration of a 300-µg bolus SST, one terminally ill patient experienced paraplegia and anesthesia, from which he recovered within 20 h. The analgesic effect of SST started prior to the toxic effects, but lasted only for 48 min (Madrazo et al. 1987). Nevertheless, Penn et al. (1990) intrathecally infused ocreotide, an SST analogue, in five patients with cancer pain, whom he was not able to treat satisfactorily with morphine. All patients obtained adequate pain relief at a daily dose of 120–480 µg ocreotide over a period of 9–66 days without suffering severe side effects.

Discussion

There is no doubt that SST has analgesic potency, despite the fact that the underlying mechanisms are not quite clear. SST seems to lack cross-tolerance to morphine, a fact which, however, does not exclude any opioid receptor involvement in SST-induced analgesia: ϰ-opioid receptor agonists such as pentazocine and ketozocine, for example, are not able to inhibit thermal nociception. None of the patients wo have been treated so far with spinal SST underwent postmortem histological evaluation to rule out toxic damage to neurons. Moreover, all except one patient were treated with low dosages over a short period. The doses administered in animals were relatively speaking much higher, and the results of bioassays give clear evidence that SST-induced neurotoxicity is correlated with dosages and duration of the treatment. In accordance with this, severe toxicity was observed in the one patient who received a high dose of SST.

All reports failed to demonstrate that SST really had a superior analgesic effect to morphine. It is debatable whether it is really of any relevance that with SST there is absence of sedation and of other central effects of morphine. With morphine, these side effects usually cause only minor problems if the drug ist used properly.

With regard to the toxicity demonstrated in animals, extensive toxicological animal studies and thereafter preclinical studies need to be conducted to explore systematically the analgesic and possibly toxic effects of SST. We must be certain that the observed antinociceptive effects are not merely due to the generally toxic effect which SST has on many populations of neurons, but is rather specific to those neurons involved in pain transmission.

In conclusion, SST cannot be recommended for routine use as a spinal analgesic for the treatment of either acute or chronic pain at present.

References

Chrubasik J, Meynadier J, Blond S, et al. (1984) Somatostatin, a potent analgesic. Lancet ii:1208–1209

Chrubasik J, Meynadier J, Scherpereel P, Wünsch E (1985) The effect of epidural somatostatin on postoperative pain. Anesth Analg 64/11:1085–1088

Dirksen R, Lerou J, Nijhuis GM, Booij LH, Jurna I (1990) Intrathecal somatostatin produces effects dependent on the interval between catheter implantation and drug injection. Life Sci 47/14:1347–1354

Gaumann DM, Yaksh TL (1988) Intrathecal somatostatin in rats: antinociception only in the presence of toxic effects. Anesthesiology 68:733–742

Jessell TM, Dodd J (1986) Neurotransmitters and differentiation antigens in subsets of sensory neurons projecting to the spinal dorsal horn. In: Martin JB, Barches JD (eds) Neuropeptides in neurologic and psychiatric disease. Raven, New York, pp 11–133

Kuraishi Y, Hirota N, Sato Y, Hino Y, Satoh M, Takagi H (1985) Evidence that substance P and somatostatin transmit separate information related to pain in the spinal dorsal horn. Brain Res 325:294–298

Leblanc R, Gauthier S, Gauvin M, et al. (1988) Neurobehavioral effects of intrathecal somatostatinergic treatment in subhuman primates. Neurology 38:1887–1890

Madrazo I, Franco Bourland RE, Leon-Meza VM, Mena I (1987) Intraventricular somatostatin-14, arginine, vasopressin and oxytocin: analgesic effect in a patient with intractable cancer pain. Appl Neurophysiol 50:427–432

Meynadier J, Chrubasik J, Dubar M, Wuensch E (1985) Intrathecal somatostatin in terminal ill patients. A report of two cases. Pain 23/1:9–12

Ohkubo T, Shibata M, Takahashi H, Inoki R (1990) Roles of substance P and somatostatin on transmission of nociceptive information induced by formalin in spinal cord. J Pharmacol Exp Ther 252/2:1261–1268

Penn D, Paice JA, Kroix JS (1990) Intrathecal octreotide for cancer pain. Lancet 335:738

Polak JM, Bloom SR (1986) Somatostatin localization in tissues. Scand J Gastroenterol 21:11–21

Sandkühler J, Fu QG, Helmchen C (1990) Spinal somatostatin superfusion in vivo affects activity of rat nociceptive dorsal horn neurons: comparison with spinal morphine. Neuroscience 34/3:565–576

Tiseo PJ, Adler MW, Liu-Chen LY (1990) Differential release of substance P and somatostatin in the rat spinal cord in response to noxious cold and heat, effect of dynorphin A. J Pharmacol Exp Ther 252/2:539–545

Unger J, Weindl A, Ochs G, Struppler A (1988) CSF somatostatin is elevated in patients with postzoster neuralgia. Neurology 38:1423–1426

Wall PD, Woolf C (1986) The brief and the prolonged facilitatory effects of unmyelinated afferent input on the rat spinal cord are independently influenced by peripheral nerve injury. Neuroscience 17:1199–1206

Bombesin Receptor Antagonists: Different Classes and Cellular Basis of Action

R. T. Jensen, J. E. Mrozinski Jr., and D. H. Coy

National Institutes of Health, Building 10, Room 9C-103, Bethesda, MD 20892, USA

Introduction

The naturally occurring bombesin (Bn)-related peptides can be divided structurally into three different groups based on chemical structure (Erspamer 1988; Erspamer and Melchiorri 1977; Minamino et al. 1983, 1984). The amphibian peptide Bn resembles other amphibian peptides such as alytesin and the mammalian peptide gastrin-releasing peptide (GRP) (Anastasia et al. 1971; Erspamer 1988; Erspamer and Melchiorri 1977; McDonald et al. 1979) in possessing a carboxy terminal Gly-His-Leu-Met-amide (Fig. 1). The second class includes the amphibian peptides ranatensin and litorin, which resemble the mammalian peptide neuromedin B (Erspamer 1988; Erspamer and Melchiorri 1977; Minamino et al. 1983, 1984) in possessing a COOH terminal Gly-His-Phe-Met-amide (Table 1). The third group, comprised of the amphibian peptide phyllolitorin and other structurally related amphibian peptides, have at present no mammalian counterpart and are characterized by having a COOH terminal Gly-Ser-Phe-Met-amide or Gly-Ser-Leu-Met-amide (Erspamer 1988) (Table 1).

The amphibian peptides Bn and litorin, as well as the structurally related, naturally occurring mammalian peptides GRP, neuromedin B (NMB) and neuromedin C (NMC) – GRP (18–27) – (Anastasia et al. 1971; McDonald et al. 1979; Minamino et al. 1983, 1984), have been shown to have a wide range of biological or pharmacological actions (Erspamer and Melchiorri 1977; Tache et al. 1988). These include stimulation of the release of numerous gastrointestinal hormones and peptides (Ghatei et al. 1982; Kaneto et al. 1978), stimulation of pancreatic enzyme secretion by various exocrine glands (Erspamer and Melchiorri 1977; Jensen et al. 1988a), chemotaxis (Ruff et al. 1985), contraction of smooth muscle (Broccardo et al. 1976; Erspamer and Melchiorri 1977; Mizrahi et al. 1982; Severi et al. 1990), effects on the central nervous system (CNS) such as thermoregulation (Brown et al. 1988), maintenance of circadian rhythm (Albers et al. 1991), inhibition of thyroid-stimulating hormone (TSH) (Rettori et al. 1992), effects on satiety (Merali et al. 1988;

Table 1. Structure of bombesin, other structurally related, naturally occurring bombesin-related agonists, and various bombesin receptor antagonists

	Amino acid sequence														
	1	2	3	4	5	6	7	8	9	10	11	12	13	14	
Agonists															
Bombesin (Bn)	pGlu	Gln	Arg	Leu	Gly	Asn	Gln	Trp	Ala	Val	Gly	His	Leu	Met	NH_2
GRP(18-27)(NMC)					–	–	His	–	–	–	–	–	–	–	–
Alytesin	–	Gly	–	–	–	Thr	–	–	–	–	–	–	–	–	–
Neuromedin B					–	–	Leu	–	–	Thr	–	–	Phe	–	–
Litorin						pGlu	–	–	–	–	–	–	Phe	–	–
Ranatensin				pGlu	Val	Pro	–	–	–	–	–	–	Phe	–	–
Phyllolitorin						pGlu	Leu	–	–	–	–	Ser	Phe	–	–
Antagonists															
[DPhe[12]]Bn	–	–	–	–	–	–	–	–	–	–	–	DPhe	–	–	–
[Leu[14], ψ9-10]Bn	–	–	–	–	–	–	–	–	$-\psi$	–	–	–	–	Leu	–
[Leu[14], ψ13-14]Bn	–	–	–	–	–	–	–	–	–	–	–	–	$-\psi$	Leu	–
[DPhe[6], Cpa[14], ψ13-14]Bn(6-14)						DPhe	–	–	–	–	–	–	$-\psi$	Cpa	–
[DPhe[6]]Bn(6-13)ethylamide						DPhe	–	–	–	–	–	–	–	$NHCH_2CH_3$	
Isobutyryl-[DAla[24]]GRP(20-26)methylamide						$(CH_3)_2CHCO$	His	–	–	–	DAla	–	–	$NHCH_3$	
[DPhe[6]]Bn(6-13) ethyl ester						DPhe	–	–	–	–	–	–	–	OCH_2CH_3	
Ac-GRP(20-26) ethyl ester						Ac	His	–	–	–	–	–	–	OCH_2CH_3	
[D-F_5-Phe[6],D-Ala[11]]Bn(6-13)methyl ester						D-F_5-Phe	–	–	–	–	DAla	–	–	OCH_3	
[DPro[4], DTrp[7,9,10]]SP(4-11)							DPro	Gln	Gln	DTrp	Phe	DTrp	DTrp	–	–
[DArg[1], DTrp[7,9]]Leu[11]]SP				DArg	Pro	Lys	Pro	Gln	Gln	DTrp	Phe	DTrp	–	Leu	–
	1	2	3	4	5	6	7	8	9	10	11	12	13	14	

The numbers at the top refer to the amino acid position from the NH_2 terminus of bombesin. Key: –, the same amino acid is in this position in the indicated peptide as in bombesin; ψ, substitution of a reduced peptide bond at the indicated site (i.e., CONH changed to CH_2NH); Bn, bombesin; NMC, neuromedin C (GRP 18-27); GRP, gastrin-releasing peptide; Ac, acetyl; Cpa, p-chlorophenylalanine; D-F_5-Phe, D-2,3,4,5,6-pentafluorophenylalanine; SP, substance P.

Tache et al. 1988), and the ability to function as a growth factor in 3T3 cells, human small-cell lung cancer cells (SCLC), rat hepatocellular tumor cells, prostatic and breast adenocarcinoma cells, and in normal bronchial epithelial and endometrial stomal cells (Bologna et al. 1989; Carney et al. 1988; Corps et al. 1985; Cuttitta et al. 1985; Endo et al. 1991; Schrey et al. 1992; Seglen et al. 1989; Tache et al. 1988; Willey et al. 1984, Woll and Rozengurt 1988; Woll et al. 1988). Bn-related peptides have been proposed to have an autocrine growth mechanism in regulating the growth of SCLC cells, because Bn receptor antagonists or anti-Bn antibodies have inhibited growth in vitro and in vivo (Cuttitta et al. 1985; Mahmoud et al. 1989; Woll and Rozengurt 1988). The physiological importance of Bn in each of the processes is presently unclear. These observations suggest that potent Bn receptor antagonists might have widespread utility, not only in resolving the role of Bn-related peptides in various physiological processes, but also possibly a clinical role as inhibitors of the growth-promoting effects of these peptides.

Recent cloning studies (Battey et al. 1991; Corgay et al. 1991; Spindel et al. 1990; Wada et al. 1991) confirm results from previous binding and functional studies (Ladenheim et al. 1990; M. C. Lee et al. 1991; Mizrahi et al. 1982; Severi et al. 1990; von Schrenck et al. 1989, 1990) that at least two classes of receptors mediate the action of Bn-related peptides. One class, the GRP-preferring receptor in the human, is a 384-amino acid peptide and has a 55% homology with the 390 amino acid, human NMB receptor (Corgay et al. 1991). Hydropathy analysis revealed each receptor has a seven-transmembrane spanning structure typical of the G protein coupled receptor superfamily (Battey et al. 1991; Corgay et al. 1991; Spindel et al. 1990; Wada et al. 1991).

In situ hybridization studies show that both receptors are widely distributed in the CNS (Battey and Wada 1991; Wada et al. 1991). Binding and functional studies have shown GRP receptors in the CNS, pituitary cells, pancreatic acinar cells and on various cell lines such as murine 3T3 fibroblasts, prostatic adenocarcinoma cells, SCLC cells and breast adenocarcinoma cells (Battey and Wada 1991; Bologna et al. 1989; Giacchetti et al. 1990; Jensen et al. 1978; Tache et al. 1988; Westendorf and Schonbrunn 1983; Zachary and Rozengurt 1985). Binding and functional studies have shown NMB receptors in the CNS, gastrointestinal smooth muscle, and various cell lines such as rat glioblastoma C-6 cells and some SCLC cells (Battey and Wada 1991; Ladenheim et al. 1990; M.C. Lee et al. 1991; Severi et al. 1990; von Schrenck et al. 1989, 1990; Wang et al. 1992). Similar to occupation of GRP receptors on 3T3 cells or SCLC cells by Bn or GRP, a recent study demonstrates occupation of NMB receptors on SCLC cells can cause growth (Moody et al. 1992). At present it is unclear which type of Bn receptor mediates which of the reported biological effects of Bn-related peptides.

Besides the development of highly selective agonists, the development of potent, selective antagonists which distinguish these two receptor classes will be important research tools in allowing answers to this question to be obtained.

In recent studies a number of different classes of Bn receptor antagonists have been identified (Coy and Jensen 1992; Coy et al. 1988, 1989, 1991, 1992; Heimbrook et al. 1989; Heinz-Erian et al. 1987; Jensen et al. 1984a; Saari et al. 1989; Valentine et al. 1992; Wang et al. 1990a, b). Some recent studies (von Schrenck et al. 1989; Wang et al. 1992) suggest that a number of these antagonists can differentiate between the two classes of Bn receptors and may be particularly useful in defining the class of Bn receptor mediating various processes. In the following sections, the recent advances in developing Bn antagonists in each of these classes of antagonists, as well as their mechanisms of action, will be reviewed.

Bn Receptor Antagonists – General

Recent studies provide evidence for five different classes of Bn antagonists. As will be reviewed under the discussion of each class of antagonists below, at least three of the classes of antagonists are known to be specific antagonists of the action of Bn. All, except for the nonpeptide antagonists, have been extensively studied and are known to be receptor antagonists which act in a competitive manner, as shown by pharmacological studies and by binding studies. Not all function as receptor antagonists in all species, with recent studies (Coy et al. 1990b; Dickinson et al. 1988; Wang et al. 1990b) suggesting that in some species a number of these compounds function as partial agonists. At present, as will be discussed further in a later section, all of the current potent Bn receptor antagonists are selective for the GRP receptor. No high affinity NMB receptor antagonists currently exist. A number of studies have provided evidence that Bn-related peptides can cause down-regulation of the Bn receptor which, in some cases, is specific for one class of Bn receptors (P.C. Lee et al. 1980; Millar and Rozengurt 1990; Swope and Schonbrun 1990). However, at present this has been used in very few systems to determine the physiological role of Bn and, therefore, while a potentially useful approach, information is too limited to discern its potential usefulness and it will thus not be discussed further.

The first class of Bn receptor antagonists, described in 1984 (Jensen et al. 1984a), functions primarily in the micromolar range (0.1–100 μM) and includes the D-amino acid substituted substance P or substance P-4-11 analogues that function as substance P-receptor antagonists (1 and 2 in Table 2). Of these, [D-Arg^1,D-Pro^2,D-Trp^{7,9},Leu^{11}]substance P, [D-Arg^1,D-Trp^{7,9},Leu^{11}]substance P (spantide) (Table 1) and [D-Arg^1,D-Phe^5,D-Trp^{7,9},Leu^{11}]substance P are three of the most potent (Coy et al. 1988; Jensen et al. 1988a; Woll and Rozengurt 1988). The second class includes analogues of Bn with D-amino acid substitutions for His^{12} (Heinz-Erian et al. 1987; Saeed et al. 1989). These peptides are more selective for Bn receptors than the D-amino acid substituted substance P analogues which function as Bn receptor antagonists, but are limited by potency (K_i, 0,3–10 μM) (3 and 4 in Table 2; Table 1) and solubility. A third class of Bn receptor antagonists include various reduced peptide bond analogues of Bn (Tables 1, 2).

Table 2. Affinities and potencies of analogues of substance P or [D-Phe^{12}]Bn and bombesin pseudopeptides for GRP receptors in different species

Peptide	Murine 3T3 cells		Pancreatic acini			
			Guinea-pig		Rat	
	IC_{50}	K_i (nM)	IC_{50} (nM)	K_i (nM)	IC_{50} (nM)	K_i (nM)
1. [D-Arg^1, D-Pro^2, D-Trp^{7,9}, Leu^{11}]SP	2 900 ± 300	5 200 ± 1 100	1 400 ± 300	8 900 ± 1 600	Agonist > 1 μM	11 323 ± 1 780
2. [D-Pro^4, D-Trp^{7,9,10}]SP(4-11)	ND	8 800 ± 800	3 400 ± 700	19 300 ± 200	Agonist > 1 μM	11 159 ± 580
3. [D-Phe^{12}, Leu^{14}]Bn	> 5 000	10 400 ± 2 000	2 000 ± 200	4 000 ± 400	> 10 000	1 300 ± 20
4. [D-Phe^{6,12}, Leu^{14}]Bn	ND	6 600 ± 1 700	300 ± 5	2 000 ± 200	> 10 000	> 10 000
5. [Leu^{14}, ψ13-14]Bn	18 ± 12	68 ± 8	35 ± 7	60 ± 6	P Agon (11% MAX)	434 ± 65
6. [Leu^{14}, ψ13-14]BN(6-14)	62 ± 18	290 ± 50	150 ± 40	330 ± 30	ND	1 101 ± 243
7. [Leu^8, ψ8-9]Litorin	335 ± 120	55 ± 5	46 ± 16	160 ± 15	Agonist	778 ± 408
8. [D-Phe^6, Leu^{14}, ψ13-14]Bn(6-14)	9 ± 4	7 ± 1	8 ± 1	14 ± 2	P Agon (11% MAX)	62
9. [D-Phe^6, Phe^{14}, ψ13-14]Bn(6-14)	1 ± 0.3	3 ± 1	8 ± 1	10 ± 2	P Agon (20% MAX)	32
10. [D-Phe^6, Cpa^{14}, ψ13-14]Bn(6-14)	1.0 ± 0.1	5 ± 1	2 ± 1	ND	10 ± 2	42 ± 5
11. [D-Phe^{6,14}, ψ13-14]Bn(6-14)	6 ± 1	12 ± 2	17 ± 3	64 ± 4	49 ± 2	97 ± 13

IC_{50} is the concentration causing half-maximal inhibition of bombesin-stimulated enzyme secretion from guinea pig or rate pancreatic acini or [^{3}H]thymidine incorporation into 3T3 cells (Coy et al. 1988, 1989, 1990b; Heinz-Erian et al. 1987; Jensen et al. 1984a); K_d values were calculated using the method of Cheng and Prusoff from inhibition of binding of 50 pM ^{125}I-[Tyr^4]Bn to either guinea pig or rat pancreatic acini (Coy et al. 1988, 1989, 1990b; Heinz-Erian et al. 1987; Jensen et al. 1988b, 1984a) or 3T3 cells (Coy et al. 1988, 1989). Abbreviations: SP, substance P; Bn, bombesin; ψ, pseudopeptide bond with insertion of CH_2NH for CONH; Cpa, chlorophenylalanine; ND, no data; P Agon (% MAX), partial agonist and the percentage of the maximal stimulation of that caused by a full agonist at a concentration of 10 μM of the indicated peptide.

Table 3. Affinities and potencies of analogues of des-Met[14] bombesin and des-Met[14] GRP for GRP receptors in different species

Peptide	Pancreatic acini					
	Murine 3T3 cells		Guinea pig		Rat	
	IC_{50} (nM)	K_i (nM)	IC_{50} (nM)	K_i (nM)	IC_{50} (nM)	K_i (nM)
1. Bn(1-13)NH_2	226 ± 70	88 ± 21	33 ± 10	216 ± 30	2 300 ± 230	296 ± 28
2. Bn(6-13)NH_2	1 600 ± 75	1 200 ± 170	610 ± 230	1 800 ± 310	5 200 ± 1400	> 10 000
3. [D-Phe[6]]Bn(6-13)NH_2	29 ± 16	23 ± 1	24 ± 11	96 ± 21	100 ± 20	27 ± 6
4. [D-Phe[6]]BN(6-13)ethylamide	0.7 ± 0.3	3.3 ± 0.1	7 ± 1	16 ± 3	30 ± 11	27 ± 5
5. [D-Phe[6]]Bn(6-13)propylamide	0.6 ± 0.2	2 ± 1	2 ± 1	6 ± 1	15 ± 2	6 ± 1
6. [D-Phe[6]]Bn(6-13)butylamide	Agonist > 1 μM	5 ± 1	P Agon (35% MAX)	28 ± 4	Agonist	14 ± 1
7. [D-Phe[6]]Bn(6-13)hexylamide	Agonist > 1 μM	6 ± 1	P Agon (15% MAX)	16 ± 2	Agonist	103 ± 8
8. [D-Phe[6]]Bn(6-12)ethylamide	> 10 000	5 000 ± 900	3 400 ± 580	6 600 ± 750	6 000 ± 1600	> 10 000
9. [D-Phe[6]]Bn(6-13)hydrazide	2 ± 1	2 ± 1	4 ± 1	5 ± 1	6 ± 1	22 ± 1
10. [D-Phe[6]]Bn(6-13)methyl ester	1 ± 0.2	1.1 ± 0.2	2 ± 1	7 ± 1	3 ± 1	10 ± 2
11. [D-Phe[6]]Bn(6-13)ethyl ester	2.4 ± 0.4	2 ± 1	1.1 ± 0.3	3 ± 1	2 ± 1	5 ± 1
12. N-Ac-GRP(20-26)methyl ester	2.5 ± 0.1	2 ± 1	4 ± 1	10 ± 1	15 ± 2	17 ± 1

IC_{50} is the concentration causing half-maximal inhibition of bombesin-stimulated enzyme secretion from pancreatic acini or [^{3}H]thymidine incorporation into 3T3 cells (Wang et al. 1990 a, b); K_i values calculated by method of Cheng and Prusoff from inhibition of binding of 50 pM ^{125}I-[Tyr^4]Bn in each of the cell systems.

Abbreviations: Bn, bombesin; GRP, gastrin-releasing peptid; Ac, acetyl; p Agon (% MAX), partial agonist and the percentage of the maximal stimulation at a concentration of 10 μM of that caused by a full agonist.

In these peptides, the CONH group of the peptide bond is either changed to CH_2NH (a ψ bond replacement) (Coy et al. 1988, 1989, 1990 b) or to CH_2O (Saari et al. 1989) or CH_2S (Edwards et al. 1992). The peptide, [Leu^{14}, ψ13-14]Bn (K_i, 60 n*M;* 5 in Table 2) was the first Bn receptor antagonist described with sufficient potency to be generally useful (Coy et al. 1988). Recent studies (Coy et al. 1989; 1990 b) have reported a number of more potent members of this class, of which the analogue [D-Phe^6,Cpa^{14},ψ13-14]Bn(6-14) (10 in Table 1) is one of the most potent. The fourth class consists of des-Met analogues of the COOH-terminus of GRP [(des-Met^{27}) GRP analogues] or of Bn [(des-Met^{14} Bn analogues)] (Camble et al. 1989; Coy et al. 1992; Heimbrook et al. 1989; Wang et al. 1990 a, b). These are the most potent and selective group of antagonists at present. Of these the most potent antagonists in vitro are [D-Phe^6]Bn(6-13)ethyl ester, Ac-GRP(20-26)methyl ester and isobutyryl-[D-Ala^{24}]GRP(20-26) methylamide (K_i, 1–10 n*M* range) (Table 3) (Camble et al. 1989; Heimbrook et al. 1989; Wang et al. 1990 a, b). In vivo the analogue [D-2,3,4,5,6-penta fluoro-Phe^6,D-Ala^{11}]Bn(6-13)methyl ester has a prolonged duration of action (Coy et al. 1992) and should, therefore, be particularly useful for studies requiring prolonged receptor blockade. The fifth class of Bn antagonists are the nonpeptide antagonists, two of which, CP-70,030 and CP-75,998, were recently described (Valentine et al. 1992). Each of these compounds had relatively low potency with IC_{50} values of 1.5–3 μM for displacing radiolabeled GRP from rat brain receptors and IC_{50} values of 1.5 ± 0.1 μM for inhibiting Bn-induced phosphoinositide turnover in rat pituitary GH_3 cells (Valentine et al. 1992). The specificity of action of these nonpeptide analogues is unknown. Because of the lack of any other data on nonpeptide Bn receptor antagonists except for these two compounds (Valentine et al. 1992), they will not be discussed further. Below, recent studies with each of these different classes of antagonists will be reviewed and the evidence that each class functions as a Bn receptor antagonist reviewed briefly.

Specific Classes of Bn Receptor Antagonists

D-Amino Acid Substituted Substance P Analogue Antagonists

The substance P receptor antagonist [D-Arg^1,D-Pro^2,D-$Trp^{7,9}$,Leu^{11}] substance P was the first member of this class described (Jensen et al. 1984 a). Subsequent studies demonstrated that numerous D-amino acid analogues of substance P or substance P-4-11, each of which functioned as a substance P receptor antagonist, also functioned as an antagonist of the action of Bn (Jensen et al. 1988 b). In one study (Jensen et al. 1988 b), each of four different substance P and two different substance P-4-11 analogues examined which functioned as a substance P receptor antagonist, also functioned as an antagonist of the action of Bn (Table 4). In this study (Jensen et al. 1988 b), it was concluded that the mechanism of the ability of these analogues to inhibit the action of Bn was by functioning as Bn receptor antagonists. This conclusion

Table 4. Comparison of the apparent affinities of agonists and antagonists for GRP receptors and substance P receptors on guinea pig pancreatic acini

	Affinity or Potency (μ*M*)				
	GRP receptor		Substance P receptor		K_i ratio[a]
	EC_{50}/IC_{50}[b]	K_i	EC_{50}/IC_{50}[b]	K_i	
Agonist					
Bn	0.0003 ± 0.0001	0.004 ± 0.001	N/A	>30	0.00001
SP	N/A	>100	0.003 ± 0.001	0.0025 ± 0.0005	$>40\,000$
SP(4-11)	N/A	>100	0.5 ± 0.01	0.14 ± 0.03	>714
Antagonist					
[D-Pro^2, D-Phe^7, D-Trp^9]SP	35	38 ± 4	11	6.5 ± 1.1	6
[D-Pro^2, D-Trp^{7,9}]SP	35	18 ± 2	3.4	1.8 ± 0.2	10
[D-Pro^4, D-Trp^{7,9}]SP(4-11)	15	35 ± 4	3.4	1.1 ± 0.2	32
[D-Pro^4, D-Trp^{7,9,10}]SP(4-11)	15	19 ± 3	1.7	1.9 ± 0.5	10
[D-Arg^1, D-Pro^2, D-Trp^{7,9}, Leu^{11}]SP	7.6	9 ± 2	1.7	1.1 ± 0.1	9
[D-Arg^1, D-Trp^{7,9}, Leu^{11}]SP	4	5 ± 1	0.7	0.5 ± 0.1	10

Data are modified from Jansen et al. 1988b. Abbreviations: SP, substance P; Bn, bombesin; SP(4-11), COOH terminal octapeptide of substance P; N/A, not applicable.

[a] K_i ratio was calculated as the affinity (K_i) of the indicated analogue for the GRP receptor divided by its affinity (K_i) for the SP receptor.

[b] Agonist activity is measured as EC_{50} stimulation, antagonist activity as IC_{50} stimulation.

was supported by a number of findings. Each substance P analogue inhibited binding of ^{125}I-[Tyr]Bn with the same relative affinity, with which it inhibited the action of Bn, whereas their affinities for occupying the substance P receptor differed from those for occupying Bn receptors (Table 4). None of the analogues increased the dissociation of bound ^{125}I-[Tyr^4]Bn; therefore, they were not functioning as pseudocompetitive antagonists. Substance P or substance P-4-11, itself, did not inhibit the action of Bn at concentrations that completely occupied the substance P receptor, suggesting that substance P receptor occupation by agonists was not, in some manner, changing Bn receptor affinity (Table 4). Pharmacological analysis of the inhibitory action of these analogues demonstrated that the substance P or substance P-4-11 analogues caused a parallel rightward shift of the dose-response curve for substance P or Bn, and the slope of the Schild plots were not significantly different from unity, as shown in Figs. 1 and 2 for one substance P analogue, [D-Arg^1,D-Pro^2,D-Trp^{7,9},Leu^{11}]SP (Jensen et al. 1984a; Zhang et al. 1988). These results with [D-Arg^1,D-Pro^2,D-Trp^{7,9},Leu^{11}] substance P are similar to that seen with the other substance P analogues which function as receptor antagonists at both substance P and Bn receptors but with different affinities. These analogues

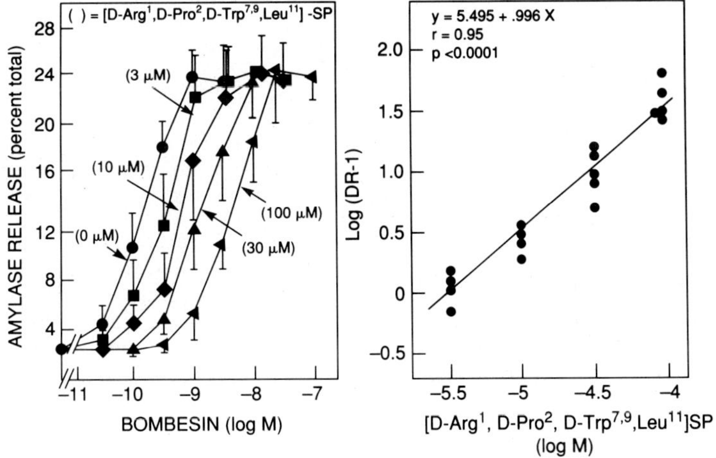

Fig. 1. Effect of various concentrations of [D-Arg^1, D-Pro^2, D-Trp^{7,9}, Leu^{11}] substance P (*SP*) on bombesin-stimulated amylase from guinea pig pancreatic acini. *Left panel,* Dispersed pancreatic acini were incubated with the concentrations of [D-Arg^1, D-Pro^2, D-Trp^{7,9}, Leu^{11}]SP, shown in parentheses with the indicated concentrations of bombesin for 30 min incubation at 37 °C. Amylase release was expressed as the percentage of total cellular amylase released during the incubation. *Right panel,* Data from left panel plotted in the form of Schild. The best fit was determined by least-squares analysis. The dose-ratio (*DR*) is the ratio of the concentration required to give half-maximal stimulation in the presence of a given concentration of [D-Arg^1, D-Pro^2, D-Trp^{7,9}, Leu^{11}]SP to the concentration required to give half maximal stimulation in the absence of [D-Arg^1, D-Pro^2, D-Trp^{7,9}, Leu^{11}]SP. The slope of the regression line (slope = 0.996) was not significantly different from unity, consistent with [D-Arg^1, D-Pro^2, D-Trp^{7,9}, Leu^{11}]SP functioning as a competitive antagonist with an affinity of 2.9 μ*M*. Data modified from Jensen et al. (1984a)

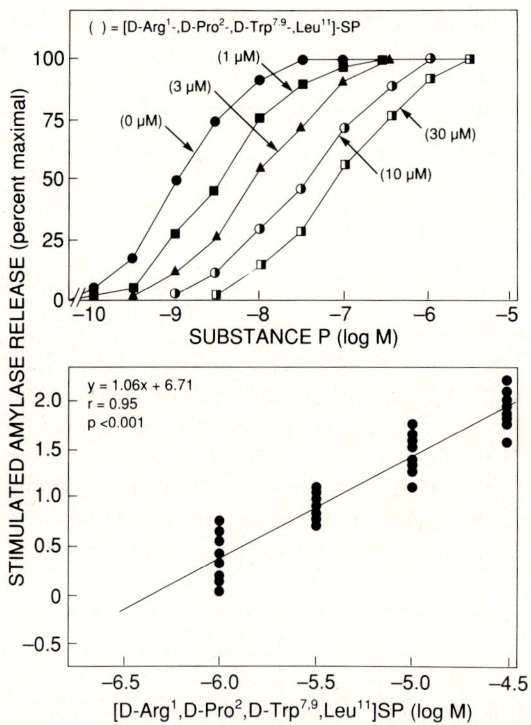

Fig. 2. Effect of various concentrations of [D-Arg^1, D-Pro^2, D-Trp^{7,9}, Leu^{11}]SP on substance P-stimulated amylase from guinea pig pancreatic acini. *Top panel,* Dispersed pancreatic acini were incubated with the concentrations of [D-Arg^1, D-Pro^2, D-Trp^{7,9}, Leu^{11}]SP, shown in parentheses with the indicated concentrations of substance P for 30 min incubation at 37 °C. Amylase release was expressed as the percentage of the stimulation caused by a maximally effective concentration of substance P (i.e., 10 n*M*). *Bottom panel,* Data from left panel plotted in the form of Schild. The best fit was determined by least-squares analysis. The dose-ratio (*DR*) is the ratio of the concentration required to give half-maximal stimulation in the presence of a given concentration of [D-Arg^1, D-Pro^2, D-Trp^{7,9}, Leu^{11}]SP to the concentration required to give half-maximal stimulation in the absence of [D-Arg^1, D-Pro^2, D-Trp^{7,9}, Leu^{11}]SP. The slope of the regression line (slope = 1.06) was not significantly different from unity consistent with [D-Arg^1, D-Pro^2, D-Trp^{7,9}, Leu^{11}]SP functioning as a competitive inhibitor of the action of substance P with an affinity of 0.47 μ*M*. Data modified from Jensen et al. (1984b)

have been reported in vitro to inhibit Bn-induced mitogenic stimulation of 3T3 cells (Rozengurt 1988), Bn-stimulated pepsinogen release from frog esophageal glands (Shirakawa and Hirschowitz 1985), and Bn-stimulated pancreatic enzyme secretion (Holst et al. 1990; Jensen et al. 1984a; Shirakawa and Hirschowitz 1985) by some investigators (Yachnis et al. 1984), but not by others (Pappas et al. 1984), to inhibit the actions of Bn in vivo. The utility of these peptides is limited by their selectivity, because each is also a substance P receptor antagonist, and furthermore some analogues also inhibit the action of vasopressin on 3T3 cells (Woll and Rozengurt 1988) or cholecystokinin in pancreatic acinar cells (Jensen et al. 1988 b; Shirakawa and Hirschowitz 1985). These analogues, in general, all have a significantly higher affinity for substance P receptors than Bn receptors (Figs. 1, 2; Table 4). Their utility is also limited by potency because these substance P analogues function as Bn receptor antagonists only in the micromolar range (1 and 2 in Table 2; Table 4). Therefore, in vivo, their possible widespread utility is significantly limited.

D-Amino Acid^{12} Bn Analogue Antagonists

Numerous D-amino acid substituted analogues of Bn have been synthesized; however, only various D-amino acid^{12} analogues of Bn have been described to function as antagonists (Heinz-Erian et al. 1987; Rivier and Brown 1978; Saeed et al. 1989). These studies combined with the original studies of Broccardo et al. (1976) which demonstrated that Trp^{8} and His^{12} of Bn were essential amino acids in Bn for biological activity, suggest that substitutions in these positions might be particularly important in determining agonist or antagonist activity. In one study (Saeed et al. 1989) a number of substitutions in position 12 of Bn such as D-Phe, D-chlorophenylalanine, and D-Tyr, but not L-Phe, D-pyridylalanine (D-Pal), D-Trp, D-Arg, or D-β-naphthylalanine (D-Nal) resulted in receptor antagonists, with the most potent being [D-Phe^{12}]Bn (K_i, 5–6 μM; 3 in Table 1). Attempts to increase potency by additional amino acid replacements improved potency only threefold with the [D-Phe^{6,12}]Bn analogue being the most potent (4 in Table 1) (Saeed et al. 1989). A number of findings confirm that these [D-Phe^{12}]Bn analogues are functioning as Bn receptor antagonists. Pharmacological studies demonstrated that [D-Phe^{12}]Bn analogues caused a parallel-rightward shift of the dose-response curve for Bn-stimulated amylase release from pancreatic acini, and when the data was plotted in the form of Schild the slope was not different from unity, as shown in Fig. 3 for [D-Phe^{12},Leu^{14}]Bn (Battey and Wada 1991). Furthermore, there was a close correlation between the ability of various [Phe^{12}]Bn analogues to occupy the Bn receptor (assessed by inhibiting binding of [^{125}I-Tyr^{4}]Bn) and inhibit biological activity, demonstrating that these agents functioned as receptor antagonists (Heinz-Erian et al. 19897; Saeed et al. 1989) (Table 1). Whereas these analogues have the advantage over substance P analogues in being selective for Bn receptors and not interacting with substance P receptors in some (Heinz-Erian et al. 1987) but not other tissues (Merali et al. 1988), general utility of these analogues is limited by their low solubility and potency and, therefore, they have not been generally useful for in vivo studies.

Reduced Peptide Bond (Pseudopeptide) Bn Analogue Antagonists

It was originally observed that changing the CONH peptide bond in various locations in the COOH terminus of gastrin (Martinez et al. 1985) to a reduced peptide bond of CH_2NH resulted in some analogues which functioned as

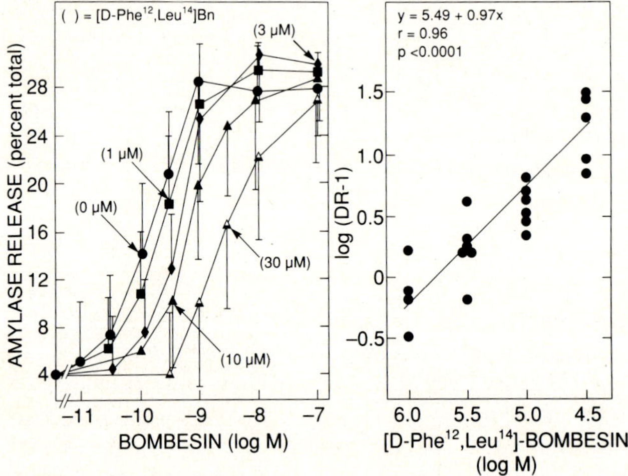

Fig. 3. Effect of various concentrations of [D-Phe^{12}, Leu^{11}]bombesin on bombesin-stimulated amylase from guinea pig pancreatic acini. *Left panel,* Dispersed pancreatic acini were incubated with the concentrations of [D-Phe^{12}, Leu^{11}]bombesin, shown in parentheses with the indicated concentrations of bombesin for 30 min incubation at 37 °C. Amylase release was expressed as the percentage of total cellular amylase released during the incubation. *Right panel,* Data from left panel plotted in the form of Schild. The best fit was determined by least-squares analysis. The dose-ratio (*DR*) is the ratio of the concentration required to give half-maximal stimulation in the presence of a given concentration of [D-Phe^{12}, Leu^{11}]bombesin to the concentration required to give half-maximal stimulation in the absence of [D-Phe^{12}, Leu^{11}]bombesin. The slope of the regression equation (slope = 0.97) was not significantly different from unity consistent with [D-Phe^{12}, Leu^{14}]bombesin functioning as a competitive antagonist with an affinity of 2.1 μ*M*. Data modified from Heinz-Gian et al. (1987)

gastrin receptor antagonists. Similar results were obtained with substance P, secretin, and growth hormone-releasing factor (Haffar et al. 1991; Hocart et al. 1990; Qian et al. 1989) and a similar strategy was applied to Bn (Coy et al. 1988, 1989, 1990b). When each peptide bond CONH group in the COOH terminal octapeptide of Bn (Coy et al. 1988) was replaced one at time by a CH_2NH group, it was found that four of the pseudopeptides were agonists with relative potencies: [Leu^{14}]Bn $= \psi$10-11 $\gg \psi$11-12 $> \psi$12-13 $> \psi$8-9, whereas two pseudopeptides were antagonists with potencies ψ13-14 $> \psi$9–10. The [Leu^{14}, ψ13-14]Bn analogue (5 in Table 1) was the first Bn antagonist (Coy et al. 1988) with affinity less than 0.1 μ*M* and was more than 50 times more potent than the [D-Phe^{12}]Bn or D-amino acid substituted substance P analogues in studies in 3T3 cells or in guinea pig pancreatic acini (Table 2) (Coy et al. 1988). [Leu^{14}, ψ13-14]Bn has been shown to inhibit in vitro Bn-stimulated pancreatic enzyme secretion, [^{3}H]thymidine incorporated and autocrine growth in 3T3 cells and various SCLC cells and in vivo to inhibit Bn-stimulated gastric acid secretion, gastrin release and increased gastric motility (Holst et al. 1990; Rossowski et al. 1989; Trepel et al. 1988; Woll et al. 1988).

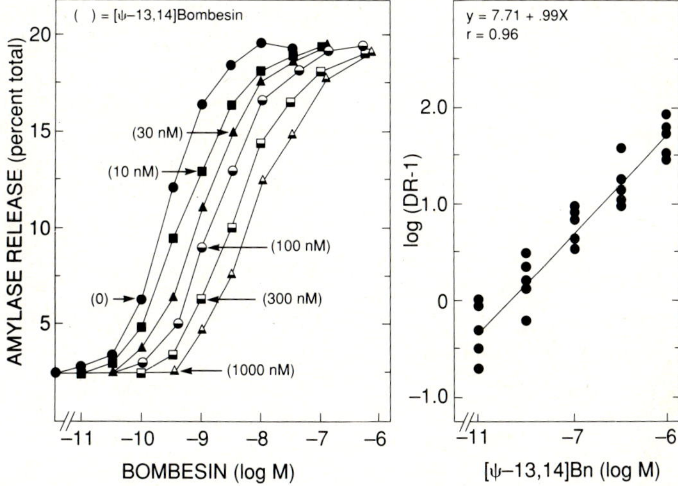

Fig. 4. Effect of various concentrations of [ψ 13,14]bombesin on bombesin-stimulated amylase from guinea pig pancreatic acini. *Left panel,* Dispersed pancreatic acini were incubated with the concentrations of [ψ 13,14]bombesin, shown in parentheses with the indicated concentrations of bombesin for 30 min incubation at 37 °C. Amylase release was expressed as the percentage of total cellular amylase released during the incubation. *Right panel,* Data from left panel plotted in the form of Schild. The best fit was determined by least-squares analysis. The dose-ratio (*DR*) is the ratio of the concentration required to give half-maximal stimulation in the presence of a given concentration of [ψ 13,14]bombesin to the concentration required to give half-maximal stimulation in the absence of [ψ 13,14]bombesin. The slope of the regression equation (slope = 0.99) was not significantly different from unity consistent with [ψ 13,14]bombesin functioning as a competitive antagonist with an affinity of 16 n*M*. Data modified from Coy et al. (1988)

A number of results demonstrated that [Leu^{14}, ψ13-14]Bn as well as other pseudopeptide analogues were inhibiting the action of Bn by functioning as Bn receptor antagonists (Coy et al. 1988, 1989, 1990 b). Studies of a number of different pseudopeptides in 3T3 cells and guinea pig pancreatic acini demonstrated a close correlation between the ability of these pseudopeptides to inhibit the action of Bn and occupy the Bn receptor (Coy et al. 1988, 1989, 1990 b). Pharmacological studies demonstrated that analogues such as [Leu^{14}, ψ13-14]Bn (Fig. 4) caused a parallel-rightward shift of the Bn-stimulated amylase release curve from pancreatic acini and that the data plotted in the form of Schild gave a slope not different from unity, suggesting competitive antagonism characteristics of a receptor antagonist (Coy et al. 1988, 1989).

A more recent study (Coy et al. 1991) has identified short-chain pseudopeptide Bn receptor antagonists that are more potent than [Leu^{14}, ψ13-14]Bn, have fewer proteolytic degradation sites, and can be more easily synthesized (Table 2). In previous studies Bn(8-14) or GRP(21-27) had been shown to be minimal COOH terminal fragment to have biological activity (Broccardo et al. 1976; Heimbrook et al. 1988), even though it had low affinity, whereas the nonapeptide Bn(6-14) has almost equal affinity to native Bn (Broccardo et al. 1976; Heimbrook et al. 1988). The formation of the nonapeptide pseudopeptide of Bn (6 in Table 2) resulted in an antagonist, but with a marked decrease in potency compared to [Leu^{14},ψ13-14]Bn (5 in Table 2). However, the ψ8-9 pseudopeptide of the Bn-related peptide, litorin (7 in Table 2), had only a minimal loss in potency. Litorin differs from Bn(6-14) in having a p-Glu in the 6 position of Bn (Fig. 1) and a Phe in the 13 position (Table 1). Because the insertion of a D-Phe^6 in the [D-Phe^{12}]Bn antagonist increased affinity (Saeed et al. 1989) and because litorin has equal affinity to Bn for GRP receptors, a similar insertion was made in the Bn nonapeptide pseudopeptide (8 in Table 2), which resulted in an antagonist with 50-fold higher affinity. The insertion of Phe, D-Phe or Cpa in position 14 (9–11 in Table 2) increased potency an additional fivefold in 3T3 cells and guinea pig pancreatic acini, resulting in antagonists with affinity in the 3–10 n*M* range (Coy et al. 1989, 1990b). Additional studies demonstrated, with the pseudopeptides as well as des-Met^{14} Bn analogues (Coy et al. 1989, 1991), that insertion of groups in the 6 position of Bn more hydrophobic than D-Phe such as D-Nal, or more hydrophilic such as D-Pal, or the insertion of other aromatic groups such as D-Trp, D-Tyr and even nonaromatic D-amino acids such as D-Leu, but not L-amino acids such as L-Phe, resulted in minimal loss of antagonist potency. In the pseudopeptide, the replacement of the COOH terminal NH_2 with OH or the further shortening of the chain length to Bn(7-14) in the pseudopeptide markedly reduced affinity. A recent study (Saari et al. 1989) demonstrates that a reduced peptide bond analogues with CONH changed to CH_2O also results in analogues with even higher affinity. One such analogue (Saari et al. 1989) Ac-[ψCH_2O 25-26]GRP(20-27) had an affinity of 30 n*M* for 3T3 cells and removal of the terminal carbamoyl group resulted in an analogue with a potency of 10 n*M* for 3T3 cells (Saari et al. 1989).

Des-Met^{14} Bn or Des-Met^{27} GRP Analogue Antagonists

In structure function studies of cholecystokinin or gastrin (Martinez et al. 1984; Spanarkel et al. 1983) it was found that the removal of the COOH terminal amino acid Phe and the formation of des-Phe amidated analogue resulted in potent antagonists and partial agonists. A similar strategy has been applied to Bn or GRP by a number of investigators (Camble et al. 1984; Coy et al. 1992; Heimbrook et al. 1989; Saari et al. 1989; Wong et al. 1990a, b) (Table 1). The analogues Ac-GRP(20-26)NH_2, Ac-GRP(18-26)NH_2, and Bn(1-13)NH_2 (1 in Table 3) were all shown to function as weak Bn receptor antagonists in 3T3 cells or guinea pig pancreatic acini (Heimbrook et al. 1989; Wang et al. 1990a). Similar to the pseudopeptides, shortening of the chain length of Bn to the nanopeptide (2 in Table 3) significantly reduced potency, but insertion of a [Phe^6] in the nanopeptide increased potency more than 20-fold (3 in Table 3) (Coy et al. 1989; Wang et al. 1990a). The formation of alkylamides (4–7 in Table 3) also increased potency with the relative potencies of the various alkylamides in 3T3 cells or guinea pig pancreas being: propyl > ethyl ≃ butyl, hexyl > heptyl. The combination of a D-Phe^6 and a COOH terminal alkylamide resulted in a number of Bn analogues with affinity in the nanomolar range (4–7 in Table 3) (Wang et al. 1990a). Similar results were obtained with GRP analogues Ac-[D-Ala^{24}]-GRP(20-26) methylamide or Ac-GRP(20-26) ethylamide reported to have affinities from 20–50 n*M* for 3T3 cells (Camble et al. 1989; Heimbrook et al. 1989). Removal of a penultimate and the terminal COOH amino acid forming a Bn(6-12) amide analogue markedly reduced potency (8 in Table 3). The formation of des-Met^{14}Bn or des-Met^{27} GRP esters or hydrazides also results in potent antagonists of the action of Bn at GRP receptors in each cell system (9–12 in Table 3). A number of results demonstrated that the various des-Met analogues were inhibiting the action of Bn by functioning as Bn receptor antagonists. For both the des-Met alkylamide and ester analogues, there was a very close correlation between their abilities to occupy the Bn receptor and to inhibit Bn-stimulated changes in cellular function (Wang et al. 1990a, b). Pharmacological studies, such as those shown in Fig. 5 for [D-F$_5$-Phe^6,D-Ala^{11}]Bn(6-13)methyl ester, demon-

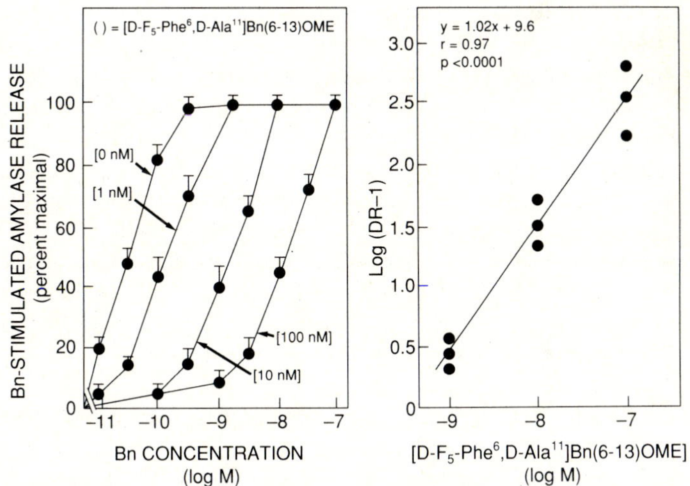

Fig. 5. Effect of various concentrations of [D-F$_5$-Phe^6, D-Ala^{11}]Bn(6-13)OME on bombesin-stimulated amylase from rat pancreatic acini. *Left panel,* Dispersed pancreatic acini were incubated with the concentrations of [D-F$_5$-Phe^6, D-Ala^{11}]Bn(6-13)OME, shown in parentheses with the indicated concentrations of bombesin for 30 min incubation at 37 °C. Amylase release was expressed as the percentage of the stimulation caused by a maximally effective concentration of bombesin alone (i.e., 10 n*M*). *Right panel,* Data from left panel plotted in the form of Schild. The best fit was determined by least-squares analysis. The dose-ratio (*DR*) is the ratio of the concentration required to give half-maximal stimulation in the presence of a given concentration of [D-F$_5$-Phe^6, D-Ala^{11}]Bn(6-13)OME to the concentration required to give half-maximal stimulation in the absence of [D-F$_5$-Phe^6, D-Ala^{11}]Bn(6-13)OME. The slope of the regression equation (slope = 1.02) was not significantly different from unity consistent with [D-F$_5$-Phe^6, D-Ala^{11}]Bn(6-13)OME functioning as a competitive antagonist with an affinity of 0.4 n*M*. Data modified from Coy et al. (1992)

strated a parallel rightward shift of the dose-response curve for Bn-stimulated amylase release which, when plotted in the form of Schild, gave a slope not different from unity demonstrating competitive antagonism (Wang et al. 1990a, b). Furthermore, des-Met analogues which functioned as partial agonists partially inhibited Bn-stimulated amylase release, demonstrating that they were interacting with the same receptor as Bn. This conclusion was further confirmed by demonstrating other analogues which functioned as Bn receptor antagonists inhibited their partial agonist activity (Wang et al. 1990b).

The fact that the formation of des-Met Bn analogues resulted in antagonists has led to the conclusion (Heimbrook et al. 1989; Wang et al. 1990a) that, similar to cholecystokinin and gastrin-related peptides, the COOH terminal amino acid of Bn-related peptides is important for initiating a biological response, but not essential for determining receptor affinity.

At present the various ester antagonists listed in Table 3 are the most potent GRP receptor antagonists in vitro (10–12 in Table 3). Ester analogues such as [D-Phe^{6}]Bn(6-13) ethyl ester (Wang et al. 1990b), Ac-GRP(20-26)ethyl ester (Heimbrook et al. 1989) and trimethyl acetyl-[D-Ala^{24}]GRP(20-26) methyl ester (Camble et al. 1989) are all potent Bn antagonists in vitro. Various des-Met Bn or GRP analogues are also potent inhibitors in vivo of Bn- or GRP-stimulated amylase release or gastrin release (Camble et al. 1989; Coy et al. 1990a, Varga et al. 1991). Recent studies have described important modifications that increase the duration of action of antagonist activity in vivo (Camble et al. 1989; Coy et al. 1992). Substitution of a [D-Ala^{24}] in GRP(20-26)methyl amide (Camble et al. 1989) or [D-Ala^{11}] in [Phe^{6}]Bn(6-13)methyl amide (Coy et al. 1992) did not significantly decrease affinity and increased the duration of inhibitory activity in vivo. The further addition of a lipophilic group to the NH_2 terminus has greatly increased in vivo potency with the peptide [D-2,3,4,5,6-pentafluoro-Phe^{6},D-Ala^{11}]Bn(6-13)methyl ester having inhibitory activity up to 4–5 h after a single bolus injection (Coy et al. 1992).

Determinants of Agonist/Antagonist Activity for Bn/GRP-Related Peptides

Figure 6 summarizes the importance of the COOH terminal dipeptide amide in determining the ability of Bn- or GRP-related peptides to bind to the GRP receptor and alter cellular function. When it was discovered that replacement of either the 9-10 or 13-14 peptide bonds of Bn by a reduced peptide bond resulted in an antagonist (Coy et al. 1988), it was suggested that this might be explained by assuming that Bn has a β-turn between Val^{10} and Leu^{14}. This was supported by previous structural studies by some (Coy and Jensen 1992; Rivier and Brown 1978) but not others (Erne and Schwyzer 1987). Such a configuration had been proposed for both somatostatin and luteinizing hormone releasing hormone (Coy et al. 1988; Van Binst and Tourwe 1992). A number of results from recent studies on Bn-related peptides support this proposed configuration. In various structure function studies, alterations of both the NH_2

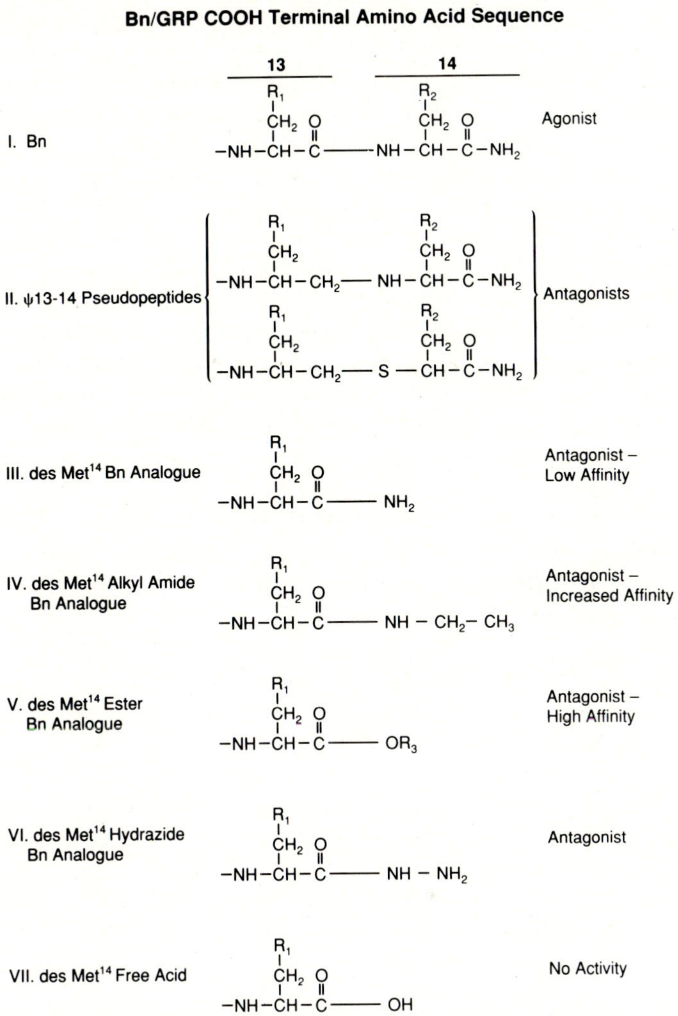

Bn/GRP COOH Terminal Amino Acid Sequence

13 — 14

I. Bn — $-NH-CH(CH_2R_1)-C(=O)-NH-CH(CH_2R_2)-C(=O)-NH_2$ — Agonist

II. ψ13-14 Pseudopeptides — $-NH-CH(CH_2R_1)-CH_2-NH-CH(CH_2R_2)-C(=O)-NH_2$; $-NH-CH(CH_2R_1)-CH_2-S-CH(CH_2R_2)-C(=O)-NH_2$ — Antagonists

III. des Met[14] Bn Analogue — $-NH-CH(CH_2R_1)-C(=O)-NH_2$ — Antagonist – Low Affinity

IV. des Met[14] Alkyl Amide Bn Analogue — $-NH-CH(CH_2R_1)-C(=O)-NH-CH_2-CH_3$ — Antagonist – Increased Affinity

V. des Met[14] Ester Bn Analogue — $-NH-CH(CH_2R_1)-C(=O)-OR_3$ — Antagonist – High Affinity

VI. des Met[14] Hydrazide Bn Analogue — $-NH-CH(CH_2R_1)-C(=O)-NH-NH_2$ — Antagonist

VII. des Met[14] Free Acid — $-NH-CH(CH_2R_1)-C(=O)-OH$ — No Activity

Fig. 6. Summary of COOH-terminal modifications of Bn or GRP that are responsible for GRP receptor agonist or antagonist activity. In *I*, the 13 and 14 refer to the two carboxyl terminal amino acids (Leu-Met-amide) of Bn or GRP which, when included in the Bn or GRP COOH terminal hexapeptide, function as potent agonists (Table 5). *II*, Formation of reduced peptide bonds in the 13-14 peptide bond (–CO–NH– to CH_2NH or CH_2SH–) results in Bn or GRP pseudopeptide analogues which function as antagonists (Table 2; Fig. 4). *III*, Des-Met[14] and des-Met[27] GRP amidated analogues function as weak antagonists of GRP receptors (Table 3). *IV*, Des-Met[14] or des-Met[27] GRP alkylamide analogues function as more potent antagonists (Table 3). *V*, Des-Met[14]Bn or des Met[27] GRP esters function as potent, highly selective antagonists in all species examined (Table 3, Fig. 5). *VI*, Des-Met[14]Bn hydrazides function as potent antagonists (Table 3). *VII*, Des-Met[14]Bn analogue is a very weak antagonist or inactive. Data modified from Coy and Jensen (1992), Coy et al. (1988, 1989), and Wang et al. (1990 a, b)

and COOH terminus of Bn analogues functioning as antagonists and markedly altered their receptor affinities, suggesting both were important in receptor interaction (Coy et al. 1989; Wang et al. 1990 b). Cyclic analogues of Bn(6-14), joined by either a disulfide bond or head-to-tail peptide bond, functioned as Bn receptor agonists (Coy et al. 1991; Knight et al. 1990). Insertion of a D-Ala^{11} into the cyclized peptide increased receptor affinity, suggesting the presence of a type II β-bond which is known to be stabilized by this modification (Coy et al. 1991). Recent molecular modeling studies further supported this configuration, suggesting that the hydrophilic side chains of the critically important amino acids (Trp^8, Val^9, Leu^{11}) might form a hydrophobic pocket projecting above the plane of the molecular and thus are crucial for determining binding affinity (Coy and Jensen 1992). From the modeling studies, the side chain of His^{12} projects from the β-bond of the molecule and it is not in a critical binding region of the peptide chain. A recent study supports this conclusion demonstrating the His^{12} can be replaced by Tyr, Ser, or Ala with little effect on affinity (Coy and Jensen 1992).

It was proposed that because of this folding configuration due to the β-turn that hydrogen bonding was occurring between Leu^{13}-Leu^{14} CO group and the Ala^9-Val^{10} NH group which was important in maintaining a configuration that resulted in receptor activation (Coy and Jensen 1992; Coy et al. 1988, 1991; Wang et al. 1990 a). The insertion of a reduced peptide bond in the 9-10 or 13-14 position (II in Fig. 6) disrupted this hydrogen bonding and increased rotational freedom, which allowed binding to the receptor to occur but without receptor activation (Coy et al. 1988). This conclusion was further supported by the results from des-Met^{14} analogues of Bn (III–VII in Fig. 6). The complete removal of the Met^{14} from Bn resulted in a series of Bn analogues that could function as Bn receptor antagonists without causing receptor activation (Wang et al. 1990 a, b). Lack of participation of the 13-14 peptide bond NH group in hydrogen bonding is also suggested by the potent antagonist activity of analogues with CH_2O or CH_2S replacements in the 13-14 position (II b in Fig. 6) (Edwards et al. 1992; Saari et al. 1989).

It was also proposed (Wang et al. 1990 a) that the ability of the addition of alkyl groups to position 13 (III in Fig. 6; Table 3) to markedly increase antagonist potency may be due to the electron-releasing properties of the alkyl substitutions, perhaps by enhancing Bn/GRP receptor interaction by enhancing hydrogen bonding. Recent studies support this conclusion (Heimbrook et al. 1989; Wang et al. 1990 b), because formation of des-Met^{14} Bn or des-Met^{27} GRP analogues with other electron-releasing groups, esters (10–12 in Table 3; III–VI in Fig. 6) or hydrazides (9 in Table 2; VI in Fig. 6) are very potent Bn receptor antagonists. In contrast, des-Met^{11} analogues such as the free acid (VII in Fig. 6) have low affinity, because electrons are distributed over two oxygen groups which decreases hydrogen bonding (Wang et al. 1990 a).

Studies have demonstrated that the COOH terminal heptapeptide of Bn or GRP was not only the minimal fragment that interacted with Bn receptor, it was also the minimal fragment with biological activity (Broccardo et al. 1976; Heimbrook et al. 1988). In some cell systems (Broccardo et al. 1976; Erspamer and Melchiorri 1977), but not others (Jensen et al. 1988 a), the COOH terminal nanopeptide was the minimal fragment equipotent Bn or GRP. Studies of both pseudopeptide Bn or GRP analogues as well as des-Met^{14} Bn or des-Met^{27} GRP analogues have led to the conclusion that the COOH terminal methionine was essential in determining biological activity, but not in determining affinity for the receptor (Coy et al. 1989; Heimbrook et al. 1989; Wang et al. 1990 a, b). Recent studies demonstrate that Met^{14} per se is not essential for biological activity, because various Bn analogues with Phe^{14}, Leu^{14}, or Nle^{14} all have agonist activity (Saeed et al. 1989). Recent studies investigating the biological activity of Bn/GRP pseudopeptides or des-Met^{14} Bn or des-Met^{27} GRP analogues (Coy et al. 1990 b; Wang et al. 1990 b) suggest that the determinants of biological activity are much more complicated than previously thought.

In the case of pseudopeptides and COOH terminal des-Phe amidated analogues of cholecystokinin or gastrin (Martinez et al. 1984; Sparnakel et al. 1983), it was reported that a number of these analogues could have partial agonist activity in some species and not others. In early studies (Coy et al. 1988; Heinz-Erian et al. 1987; Marki et al. 1981; Rivier and Brown 1978; Saeed et al. 1989) of more than 150 Bn analogues examined, no analogues with potent partial agonist activity were reported. However, a recent study (Dickinson et al. 1988) reported weak partial agonist activity in frog esophageal peptic cells with [Leu^{14}, ψ13-14]Bn, which is a relatively potent Bn antagonist in 3T3 cells or guinea pig pancreatic acini (Coy et al. 1988), suggesting that partial agonist activity might be a problem with some classes of purported Bn receptor antagonists in some species. In almost all cases, the various classes of Bn receptor antagonists were initially tested in only 3T3 cells or in guinea pig pancreatic acini and therefore data in other species or cell systems was limited. In recent studies (Coy et al. 1990 b; Wang et al. 1990 b) the ability of a number of potent Bn antagonists identified by studies in guinea pig pancreatic acini were compared to their interaction with Bn receptors in 3T3 cells as well as in rat pancreatic acini. Rat pancreatic acini were included because recent studies with cholecystokinin-related peptides suggested that for the cholecystokinin receptor, the peptide structural requirements for causing biological activity were much less stringent than in the guinea pig. In comparative studies (Coy et al. 1990 b; Wang et al. 1990 b), of 32 various Bn pseudopeptides or des-Met^{14} Bn and des-Met^{27} GRP analogues, in 3T3 cells or guinea pig pancreas there was a very close corelation in the peptide structural determinants of biological activity, but not with rat pancreatic acini. Results with a few of these analogues are summarized in Tables 2 and 3. Of the 11 substance P or Bn or GRP pseudopeptide analogues in Table 2, and 11 des-Met^{14}Bn or des-Met^{27} GRP analogues in Table 3, two had partial agonist activity in guinea pig pancreas (6 and 7 in Table 3), whereas the remaining 22 were receptor antagonists. In contrast, in rat pancreatic acini, 11 of the 20 analogues tested were Bn receptor agonists or partial agonists, whereas the others were antagonists. In general, results with 3T3 cells were similar to those seen with guinea pig pancreatic acini (Wang et al. 1990 b). These results were representative of those with all the analogues investigated in the above studies (Coy et al. 1990b; Wang et al. 1990b) in that there was close agreement between whether a given analogue had agonist or antagonist activity in 3T3 cells and guinea pig pancreas but not in rat pancreas (Wang et al. 1990b). Furthermore, a number of analogues that were partial agonists in guinea pig pancreas or 3T3 cells (such as 6 and 7 in Table 3) were full agonists in rat pancreas. It was concluded (Wang et al. 1990b) that these results suggested that, similar to receptors for cholecystokinin-related peptides, the rat pancreatic Bn receptors have less stringent peptide structural requirements for activation than those on 3T3 cells or guinea pig pancreatic acini. These studies demonstrate a number of important differences in these three different cell systems which have led to the development of analogues which are antagonists in each of these systems (Coy et al. 1990b; Wang et al. 1990b). For des-Met^{14} Bn analogues, increasing the chain length of the alkylamide up to a propylamide (5 in Table 3), but not further (analogues 6 and 7 in Table 3), markedly increased potency in each cell system, however analogues with an alkyl group longer than the propylamide had partial agonist activity (6 and 7 in Table 3) (Wang et al. 1990b). All ester analogues as well as the hydrazide analogue were potent antagonists in each cell system (2–10 n*M*) (9–12 in Table 3) (Wang et al. 1990b) and were thus the most generally useful. Most of the pseudopeptides had a small degree of GRP receptor mediated partial agonist activity in rat pancreas (Coy et al. 1990b; Wang et al. 1990b), including [D-Phe^{6},Phe^{14},ψ13-14]Bn(6-14) (9 in Table 2) or [Leu^{14},ψ13-14]Bn (5 in Table 2), which had 20% and 11%, respectively, of the agonist activity of Bn. However, a recent study demonstrated that the insertion of either a Cpa^{14} or D-Phe^{14} (analogues 10 and 11 in Table 3), resulted in potent antagonists in each of the cell systems (Coy et al. 1990b). These results suggest that the des-Met^{14} Bn or des-Met^{27} GRP ester, hydrazide or propylamide analogues and the pseudopeptide analogues with Cpa^{14} or D-Phe^{14} (10 and 11 in Table 3) at present may be the most universal antagonists.

Differentiation of Bn Receptor Subtypes by Various Bn Receptor Antagonists

As pointed out in the introduction, two different classes of Bn receptors have now been cloned, the GRP receptor and the NMB receptor, and found to exist widely in both the CNS and the gastrointestinal tract (Battey et al. 1991; Corgay et al. 1991; Spindel et al. 1990; Wada et al. 1991). In Table 5 the affinities and potencies are summarized of various agonists and a representative member of the various classes of antagonists for these two classes in various rat tissues. Rat pancreatic acinar cells possess only GRP receptors (von Schrenck et al. 1989, 1990), whereas rat glioblastoma C-6 tumor cells (C-6 cells) and rat esophageal muscularis mucosa possess NMB receptors (von Schrenck et al. 1989; 1990; Wada et al. 1991; Wang et al. 1992). The naturally occurring Bn-related peptides all functioned as an agonist at both receptors. For GRP receptors, litorin, ranatensin, and Bn (I.1, I.2 and I.3 in Table 5) had equally high affinity (K_i, 2–6 n*M*; EC_{50}, 0.2 n*M*), were twofold more potent

Table 5. Comparison of the affinities and potencies of various bombesin receptor agonists and antagonists for GRP

Peptide	Affinity (n*M*)				
	GPR receptor			NMB receptor	
	Rat pancreas		Rat C-6 cells	Rat esophageal muscularis muscosa	
	EC_{50}/IC_{50} [a]	K_i	(K_i)	EC_{50}/IC_{50} [a]	K_i
I. Agonists					
1. Bombesin	0.2±0.1	4± 1	19± 2	5± 2	2 ±1
2. GRP	0.4±0.1	15± 3	500±30	39±19	30 ±4
3. GRP(18-27) (Neuromedin C)	0.4±0.2	20±12	210±20	113±30	36 ±3
4. Neuromedin B	6 ±1	350±28	2± 1	4± 1	0.30±0.03
5. Litorin	0.4±0.1	6± 1	3± 1	ND	0.1 ±0.01
6. Ranatensin	0.2±0.1	2± 1	8± 1	ND	0.3 ±0.03
II. Antagonists					
1. [D-Arg[1] D-Trp[7,9], Leu[11]]SP	Agonist > 1 μ*M*	11 320±1 780	3 980± 600	35 000±12 000	9 800± 100
2. [Tyr[4], D-Phe[12]]Bn	>10 000	13 000±2 000	3 300± 200	11 000± 3 000	3 000±1 000
3. [Leu[14], ψ13-14]Bn	P Agonist (11% MAX)	434± 65	13 160± 1 782	none at 30 μ*M*	44 000±2 000
4. [D-Phe[6], Cpa[14], ψ13-14]BN(6-14)	10±2	42± 5	2 540± 1 000	none at 1 μ*M*	58 000±4 000
5. Ac-GRP(20-26)ethyl ester	15±2	17± 1	37 600±17 000	none at 1 μ*M*	52 000±5 000
6. [D-Phe[6]]Bn(6-13)ethyl ester	2±1	5± 1	2 460± 300	none at 1 μ*M*	50 000±8 000
7. [D-F_5-Phe[6]]Bn(6-13)methyl ester	0.6±0.1	5± 1	614± 110	ND	ND

[a] Agonist activity is expressed as EC_{50} stimulation caused by a maximally effective concentration of Bn or NMB. Antagonist activity is expressed as IC_{50} of bombesin-stimulated enzyme secretion from pancreatic acini or muscle concentration for rat esophageal muscularis mucosa using half-maximally effective concentration of bombesin. Results partially from Coy et al. (1990a, b, 1992), Van Binst and Tourwe (1992), von Schrenck et al. (1989, 1990) and Wang et al. (1990b).

Abbreviations: GRP, gastrin-releasing peptide; Bn, bombesin; Ac, acetyl; Cpa, p-chlorophenylalanine; p Agonist (% MAX), partial agonist and the percentage of the maximal stimulation of that caused by a full agonist at a concentration of 10 μ*M* of the indicated peptide; none at 30 μ*M*, no inhibition of bombesin-stimulated activity at 30 μ*M* of indicated peptide, D-F_5-Phe, D-2,3,4,5,6 pentafluoro-phenylalanine; ND, no data.

than GRP or GRP(18-27)(NMC) (K_i, 15–20 nM; I.2 and I.3, Table 5) and 90-fold more potent than NMB (K_i, 350 nM; I.4 in Table 5). In contrast, for NMB receptors on C-6 cells or rat esophageal muscularis mucosa, NMB, litorin, and ranatensin had approximately equal high affinities, were fivefold more potent than Bn, and over 150-fold more potent than GRP or GRP(18-27) (Table 5; agonists). Therefore, the naturally occurring peptides could be divided into three groups depending on their relative affinities for GRP or NMB receptors. Litorin, ranatensin, and Bn have approximately equal high affinities for both GRP and NMB receptors, NMB has a more than 170-fold higher affinity for NMB receptors, whereas GRP and GRP(18-27) have a 30-fold and tenfold higher affinity for GRP receptors.

Recent studies (von Schrenk et al. 1989; Wang et al. 1992) demonstrate that a number of the various classes of Bn receptor antagonists have a markedly different affinity for the two different classes of Bn receptors (Table 5). At present, only potent GRP receptor antagonists exist, and the greatest selectivity has been developed for the GRP receptor over the NMB receptor. Specifically, [D-Phe^6]Bn(6-13)ethyl ester, Ac-GRP(20-26)ethyl ester, (D-F_5-Phe^6,D-Ala^{11}]Bn(6-13)methyl ester, [D-Phe^6,Cpa^{14},ψ13-14]Bn(6-14) and [Leu^{14},ψ13-14]Bn have a 500-, 200-, 123-, 60- and 30-fold higher affinity for GRP receptors on rat pancreatic acini or 3T3 cells than for NMB on rat glioblastoma C-6 cells or rat esophageal muscularis mucosa (von Schrenck et al. 1989; Wang et al. 1992). In contrast, [Tyr^4,D-Phe^{12}]Bn and the substance P analogue, [D-Arg^1,D-Trp^{7,9},Leu^{11}] substance P, had relatively low affinity for both classes of Bn receptors, but have a four-fold higher affinity for NMB receptors (II.1 and II.2 in Table 5). The ability of [Tyr^4,D-Phe^{12}]Bn, [D-Phe^6,Cpa^{14},ψ13-14]Bn(6-14) and the two ester analogues, but not the substance P analogue or [Leu^{14},ψ13-14]Bn to inhibit Bn-stimulated amylase release or contraction of the esophageal muscularis mucosa showed similar results to those in the binding studies (Table 5). The substance P analogue and [Leu^{14},ψ13-14]Bn had agonist activity in rat pancreas, but functioned as an antagonist in the esophagus. These results demonstrate that, at present, potent antagonists exist which can clearly distinguish the ability of Bn to mediated changes in biological activity by these two Bn receptor classes. Bn receptors involved in growth of tumors and various cells such as on 3T3 cells, SCLC cells, prostatic cancer and rat hepatocellular tumors (Bologna et al. 1989; Carney et al. 1988; Corps et al. 1985; Cuttitta et al. 1985; Rozengurt 1988; Seglen et al. 1989) are primarily GRP receptors and thus, potent selective antagonists exist. Furthermore, [D-F_5-Phe^6,D-Ala^{11}]Bn(6-13)methyl ester is both long acting in vivo and highly selective (Coy et al. 1992). In SCLC cells, recent studies (Moody et al. 1992) demonstrate that occupation of NMB receptors by agonists can also result in growth. At present no potent antagonists exist for this class and, furthermore, even though [Tyr^4,D-Phe^{12}]Bn and [D-Arg^1,D-Trp^{7,9},Leu^{11}] substance P are selective for this class, the selectivity is too low (four-fold) to be pharmacologically or clinically useful.

References

Albers HE, Liou S-Y, Stoper EG, Zoeller RT (1991) Interaction of colocalized neuropeptides: functional significance in the circadian timing system. J Neurosci 11:846–851

Anastasia A, Erspamer V, Bucci H (1971) Isolation and structure of bombesin and alytesin, two analogous active peptides from the skin of the European amphibians Bombina and Alytes. Experientia 27:166–168

Battey J, Wada E (1991) Two distinct receptors for mammalian bombesin-like peptides. Trends Neurosci 14:524–527

Battey JF, Way JM, Corjay MH, Shapira H, Kusano K, Harkins R, Wu JM, Slattery T, Mann E, Feldman RJ (1991) Molecular cloning of the bombesin/gastrin-releasing peptide receptor from Swiss 3T3 cells. Proc Natl Acad Sci USA 88:395–399

Bologna M, Festuccia C, Muzi P, Biordi L, Ciomei M (1989) Bombesin stimulates growth of human prostatic cancer cells in vitro. Cancer 63:1714–1720

Broccardo M, Falconieri-Erspamer GF, Melchiorri P, Negri L, De Castiglione R (1976) Relative potency of bombesin-like peptides. Br J Pharmacol 55:221–227

Brown MR, Carver K, Fisher LH (1988) Bombesin: central nervous system actions to affect the autonomic nervous system. Ann NY Acad Sci 547:174–182

Camble R, Lotton R, Dutta AS, Garner A, Hayward CF, Moore VE, Scholes PB (1989) *N*-isobutyryl-His-Trp-Ala-Val-D-Ala-His-Leu-NHME (ICI 216140). A potent in vivo antagonist analogue of bombesin/gastrin-releasing peptide (BN/GRP) derived from the C-terminal sequence lacking the final methionine residue. Life Sci 45:1521–1527

Carney DN, Moody T, Cuttitta F (1988) Bombesin: a potent mitogen for small cell lung cancer. Ann NY Acad Sci 547:303–309

Corgay MH, Dohrzanski DJ, Way JM, Viallet J, Shapira H, Worland P, Sausville EA, Battey JF (1991) Two distinct bombesin receptor subtypes are expressed and functional in human lung carcinoma cells. J Biol Chem 266:18771–18779

Corps AN, Rees LH, Brown KD (1985) A peptide that inhibits the mitogenic stimulation of Swiss 3T3 cells by bombesin or vasopressin. Biochem J 231:781–784

Coy DH, Jensen RT (1992) Structural analysis of ligand binding characteristics for the bombesin/gastrin-releasing peptide receptor. In: Moody TW (ed) Growth factors, peptides and receptors. Plenum, New York (in press)

Coy DH, Heinz-Erian P, Jiang N-Y, Sasaki Y, Taylor J, Moreau J-P, Wolfrey JP, Jensen RT (1988) Probing peptide backbone function in bombesin. J Biol Chem 263:5056–5060

Coy DH, Taylor JE, Jiang N-Y, Kim SH, Wang L-H, Huang SC, Moreau J-P, Gardner JD, Jensen RT (1989) Short pseudopeptide bombesin receptor antagonists with enhanced binding affinities for pancreatic acini and Swiss 3T3 cells display strong antimitotic activity. J Biol Chem 264:14691–14697

Coy DH, Taylor JE, Jiang N-Y, Wang L-H, Huang SC, Qian J-M, Moreau J-P, Jensen RT (1990a) Developing receptor antagonists of neuropeptides: the bombesin/GRP system. In: Schwartz TW, Hilsted LM, Rehfeld JF (eds) Neuropeptides and their receptors. Proceedings of the 29th Alfred Benzon symposium. Munksgaard, Copenhagen, pp 376–385

Coy DH, Wang L-H, Jiang N-Y, Jensen RT (1990b) Short chain bombesin pseuodpeptides which are potent and more general bombesin receptor antagonists. Eur J Pharmacol 190:31–38

Coy DH, Jiang N-Y, Kim SH, Moreau J-P, Lin J-T, Frucht H, Qian J-M, Wang L-H, Jensen RT (1991) Covalently-cyclized agonist and antagonist analogues on bombesin and related peptides. J Biol Chem 25:16441–16447

Coy DH, Mungan Z, Rossowski WJ, Cheng BL, Lin J-T, Mrozinski JE, Jensen RT (1992) Development of a potent bombesin receptor antagonist with prolonged in vivo inhibitory activity on bombesin-stimulated amylase and protein release in the rat. Peptides (in press)

Cuttitta F, Carney DN, Mulshine J, Moody TW, Fedorko J, Fishchler A, Minna JD (1985) Bombesin-like peptides can function as autocrine growth factors in human small-cell lung cancer cells. Nature 316:823–826

Dickinson KEJ, Uemara N, Sekar MC, McDaniel HB, Anderson W, Coy DH, Hirshowitz BI (1988) Partial agonist activity of the bombesin-receptor antagonist [Leu^{14}-psi-CH_2-NH-Leu^{13}]bombesin in frog peptic cells. Biochem Biophys Res Commun 157:1154–1158

Edwards JV, Fanger BO, Cashman EA, Eaton SR, McLean LR (1992) Amide bond substitutions and conformational restraints applied to bombesin antagonists. In: Smith JA, Rivier JE (eds) Proceedings of the 12th American peptide symposium. ESCOM Science, Leiden, The Netherlands

Endo T, Fukue H, Kanaya M, Mizunuma M, Fujii M, Yamamoto H, Tanaka S, Hashimoto M (1991) Bombesin and bradykinin increase inositol phosphates and cytosolic free Ca^{2+} and stimulate DNA synthesis in human endometrial stomal cells. J Endocrinol 131:313–318

Erne D, Schwyzer R (1987) Membrane structure of bombesin studied by infrared spectroscopy. Prediction of membrane interactions of gastrin-releasing peptide, neuromedin B and neuromedin C. Biochemistry 26:6316–6319

Erspamer V (1988) Discovery, isolation and characterization of bombesin-related peptides. Ann NY Acad Sci 547:3–9

Erspamer V, Melchiorri P (1977) Active polypeptides of the amphibian skin and their synthetic analogs. Pure Appl Chem 35:463–493

Ghatei MA, Jung RT, Stevenson JC, Hillyard CJ, Adrian TC, Lee YC, Christofides ND, Sarson DL, Nashiter K, MacIntyre I, Bloom SR (1982) Bombesin action on gut hormones and calcium in man. J Clin Endocrinol Metab 54:980–985

Giacchetti S, Gauville C, de Cremaux P, Bertin L, Berthon P, Abita J-P, Cuttitta F, Calvo F (1990) Characterization, in some human breast cancer cell lines, of gastrin-releasing peptide-like receptors which are absent in normal breast epithelial cells. Int J Cancer 46:293–298

Haffar BH, Coy DH, Hocart SJ, Chiang HCV, Jensen RT (1991) Reduced peptide bond pseudopeptide analogues of secretin: a new class of secretin receptor antagonists. J Biol Chem 266:316–322

Heimbrook DC, Boyer ME, Gorsky VM, Balishin NL, Kiefer DL, Oliff A, Rieman MW (1988) Minimal ligand analysis of gastrin-releasing peptide receptor binding and motogenesis. J Biol Chem 263:7016–7019

Heimbrook DC, Saari WS, Balishin NL, Friedman A, Moore KS, Riemen MW, Kiefer DM, Rotberg NS, Wallen JW, Oliff A (1989) Carboxy-terminal modification of a gastrin-releasing peptide derivative generates potent antagonists. J Biol Chem 264:11258–11262

Heinz-Erian P, Coy DH, Tamura M, Jones SW, Gardner JD, Jensen RT (1987) [D-Phe^{12}]bombesin analogues: a new class of bombesin receptor antagonists. Am J Physiol 252:G439–G442

Hocart SJ, Murphy WA, Coy DH (1990) Analogues of growth hormone releasing factor (1–29) amide containing the reduced peptide bond isostere in the N-terminal region. J Med Chem 33:1954–1958

Holst JJ, Harling H, Messell T, Coy DH (1990) Identification of the neurotransmitter/neuromodulator functions of the neuropeptide gastrin-releasing peptide in the porcine antrum, using the antagonist [Leu^{13}-psi-CH_2-Leu^{14}]bombesin. Scand J Gastroenterol 25:89–96

Jensen RT, Moody T, Pert CP, Rivier JE, Gardner JD (1978) Interaction of bombesin and litorin with specific membrane receptors on pancreatic acinar cells. Proc Natl Acad Sci USA 75:6139–6143

Jensen RT, Jones SW, Folkers K, Garnder JD (1984a) A synthetic peptide that is a bombesin receptor antagonist. Nature 309:61–63

Jensen RT, Jones SW, Lu Y-H, Xu J-C, Folkers K, Gardner JD (1984b) Interaction of substance P antagonists with substance P receptors on dispersed pancreatic acini. Biochim Biophys Acta 804:181–191

Jensen RT, Coy DH, Saeed ZH, Heinz-Erian P, Mantey S, Gardner JD (1988a) Interaction of bombesin and related peptides with receptors on pancreatic acinar cells. Ann NY Acad Sci 547:138–149

Jensen RT, Heinz-Erian P, Moran T, Mantey SA, Jones SW, Gardner JD (1988 b) Characterization of ability of various substance P antagonists to inhibit action of bombesin. Am J Physiol 254 [Gastrointest Liver Physiol 17]: G883–G890

Kaneto A, Kaneto T, Nakaya S, Kajinuma H, Kosaka K (1978) Effect of bombesin infused intrapancreatically on glucagon and insulin secretion. Metabolism 27: 549–553

Knight M, Burke TR, Pineda JD, Cohen SL, Mahmoud S, Moody TW (1990) Design of a cyclic bombesin analogue. In: Rivier J, Marshall G (eds) Proceedings of the 11th peptide symposium. ESCOM Science, Leiden, The Netherlands, pp 185–187

Ladenheim EE, Jensen RT, Mantey SA, McHugh PR, Moran TH (1990) Receptor heterogeneity for bombesin-like peptides in the rat antral nervous system. Brain Res 537: 233–240

Lee MC, Jensen RT, Coy DH, Moody TW (1991) Neuromedin B binds with high affinity to rat brain slices. J Mol Cell Neurosci 1: 161–167

Lee PC, Jensen RT, Gardner JD (1980) Bombesin induced desensitization of enzyme secretion in dispersed acini from the guinea pig pancreas. Am J Physiol 238: G213–G218

Mahmoud S, Palaszynski E, Fiskum G, Coy DH, Moody TW (1989) Small cell lung cancer bombesin receptors are antagonized by reduced peptide bond analogues. Life Sci 44: 367–373

Marki W, Brown M, Rivier JE (1981) Bombesin analogs: effects on thermoregulation and glucose metabolism. Peptides 2 [Suppl 2]: 169–177

Martinez J, Magnous R, Lignon MF, Laur J, Castro B, Bali J-P (1984) Synthesis and biological activity of new peptide segments of gastrin exhibiting gastrin receptor activity. J Med Chem 27: 1597–1601

Martinez J, Bali J-P, Rodriquez H, Castro B, Magous R, Laur J, Ligon HF (1985) Synthesis and biologic activity of some pseudo-peptide analogues of tetragastrin: the importance of the peptide backbone. J Med Chem 28: 1874–1879

McDonald TJ, Jornvall H, Nilsson G, Vagne M, Ghatei M, Bloom SR, Mutt V (1979) Characterization of a gastrin-releasing peptide from porcine non-antral gastric tissue. Biochem Biophys Res Commun 90: 227–233

Merali Z, Merchant CA, Crawley JN, Coy DH, Heinz-Erian P, Jensen RT, Moody TW (1988) [D-Phe^{12}]bombesin and other substance P analogues function as central bombesin receptor antagonists. Synapse 2: 228–287

Millar JBA, Rozengurt E (1990) Chronic desensitization to bombesin by progressive down-regulation of bombesin receptors in Swiss 3T3 cells. J Biol Chem 265: 12052–12058

Minamino N, Kangawa K, Matsuo H (1983) Neuromedin B: a novel bombasin-like peptide identified in porcine spinal cord. Biochem Biophys Res Commun 114: 541–548

Minamino N, Kangawa K, Matsuo H (1984) Neuromedin C: a bombesin-like peptide identified in porcine spinal cord. Biochem Biophys Res Commun 119: 14–20

Mizrahi J, Escher E, Larankas S, D'Orleans-Juste P, Regoli D (1982) Activities and antagonism of bombesin on urinary smooth muscles. Eur J Pharmacol 82: 101–105

Moody TW, Staley J, Zia F, Coy DH, Jensen RT (1992) Neuromedin B binds with high affinity, elevates cytosolic calcium and stimulates the growth of small cell lung cancer cell lines. J Pharmacol Exp Ther (in press)

Pappas T, Hamel D, Debas H, Walsh J, Tache Y (1984) Spantide: failure to antagonize bombesin-induced stimulation of gastrin secretin in dogs. Peptides 6: 1001–1003

Qian J-M, Coy DH, Jiang N-Y, Gardner JD, Jensen RT (1989) Reduced peptide bond pseudopeptide analogues of substance P: a new class of substance P receptor antagonists with enhanced specificity. J Biol Chem 264: 16667–16671

Rettori V, Pazos-Moura CC, Moura EG, Polak J, McCann SM (1992) Role of neuromedin B in control of the release of thyrotropin in hypothyroid and hyperthyroid rats. Proc Acad Sci USA 89: 3035–3039

Rivier JE, Brown MR (1978) Bombesin, bombesin analogues and related peptides: effects on thermoregulation. Biochemistry 17: 1766–1771

Rossowski WJ, Murphy WA, Jiang N-Y, Yeginsu O, Ertan A, Coy DH (1989) Effects of a novel bombesin antagonist analogue on bombesin-stimulated gastric acid secretion and growth hormone release in the pentobarbitol-anesthetized rat. Scand J Gastroenterol 24: 121–128

Rozengurt E (1988) Bombesin-induction of cell proliferation in 3T3 cells. Ann NY Acad Sci 547:277–292

Ruff M, Schiffman E, Terranova V, Pert CP (1985) Neuropeptides are chemoattractants for human cells and monocytes: a possible mechanism for metastasis. Clin Immunol Immunopathol 37:387–396

Saari WS, Heimbrook DC, Friedman A, Fischer TW, Oliff A (1989) A gastrin-releasing peptide antagonist containing a $\psi(CH_2O)$ amide bond surrogate. Biochem Biophys Res Commun 165:114–117

Saeed ZA, Huang SC, Coy DH, Jiang N-Y, Heinz-Erian P, Mantey S, Gardner JD, Jensen RT (1989) Effects of substitution in position 12 of bombesin on antagonist activity. Peptides 10:597–603

Schrey MP, Patel KV, Tezapsidis N (1992) Bombesin and glucocorticoids stimulate human breast cancer cells to produce endothelin, a paracrine mitogen for breast stomal cells. Cancer Res 52:1786–1790

Seglen PO, Skomedal H, Saeter G, Schwartze PE, Nesland JM (1989) Neuroendocrine dysdifferentiation and bombesin production in carcinogen-induced hepatocellular rat tumours. Carcinogenesis 10:21–29

Severi C, Jensen RT, Espamer V, D'Arpino, Torsoli A, Delle Fave G (1990) Different subtypes of receptors mediate the action of bombesin-related peptides on gastric smooth muscle cells. Am J Physiol 260:G683–G690

Shirakawa T, Hirschowitz BI (1985) Interaction between stimuli and their antagonists on frog esophageal peptic glands. Am J Physiol 249 [Gastrointest Liver Physiol 12]:G668–G673

Spanarkel M, Martinez J, Briet C, Jensen RT, Gardner JD (1983) Choleystokinin-27-32-amide – a member of a new class of cholecystokinin receptor antagonists. J Biol Chem 258:6476–6479

Spindel ER, Giladi E, Brehm P, Goodman RH, Segerson TP (1990) Cloning and functional characterization of a complementary DNA encoding the murine fibroblast bombesin/gastrin-releasing peptide receptor. Mol Endocrinol 4:1956–1963

Swope SL, Schonbrunn A (1990) Desensitization of islet cells to bombesin involves both down-modulation and inhibition of receptor function. Mol Pharmacol 37:758–766

Tache Y, Melchiorri P, Negri L (1988) Bombesin-like peptides in health and disease. Ann NY Acad Sci 547:1–540

Trepel JB, Moyer JD, Cuttitta F, Frucht H, Coy DH, Natale RB, Mulshine JL, Jensen RT, Sausville EA (1988) A novel bombesin receptor antagonist inhibits autocrine signals in a small cell lung cancer cell line. Biochem Biophys Res Commun 156:1383–1389

Valentine JJ, Nakanishi S, Hageman DL, Snider M, Spencer RW, Vinick FJ (1992) CP-70,030 and CP-75,998: the first non-peptide antagonists of bombesin and gastrin-releasing peptide. Bioorg Med Chem Lett 2:333–338

Van Binst G, Tourwe D (1992) Backbone modifications in somatostatin analogues: relation between conformation and activity. Peptide Res 5:8–12

Varga G, Reidelberger RD, Liehr RM, Bussjueger LJ, Coy DH, Solomon TE (1991) Efects of potent bombesin antagonist on exocrine pancreatic secretion in the rat. Peptides 12:493–497

von Schrenck T, Heinz-Erian P, Moran T, Mantey SA, Gardner JD, Jensen RT (1989) Characterization of a neuromedin B-preferring receptor in esophagus muscle: evidence for subtypes of bombesin receptors. Am J Physiol 256 [Gastrointest Liver Physiol 19]:G747–G758

von Schrenck T, Wang L-H, Coy DH, Villanueva ML, Mantey S, Jensen RT (1990) Potent bombesin receptor antagonists distinguish receptor subtypes. Am J Physiol 256:G747

Wada E, Way J, Shapira H, Kusano K, Leqacq-Verhayden AM, Coy DH, Jensen RT, Battey J (1991) cDNA cloning, characterization and brain region-specific expression of a neuromedin B-preferring bombesin receptor. Neuron 6:421–430

Wang L-H, Coy DH, Taylor JE, Jiang N-Y, Kim SH, Moreau J-P, Huang SC, Mantey S, Frucht H, Jensen RT (1990a) Desmethionine alkylamide bombesin analogues: a new class of bombesin receptor antagonists with potent antisecretory activity in pancreatic acini and antimitotic activity in Swiss 3T3 cells. Biochemistry 29:616–622

Wang L-H, Coy DH, Taylor JE, Jiang N-Y, Moreau J-P, Huang SC, Frucht H, Haffar BM, Jensen RT (1990b) Des-Met carboxyl-terminally modified analogues of bombesin function as potent bombesin receptor antagonists, partial agonists or agonists. J Biol Chem 265:1569–1570

Wang L-H, Battey JF, Wada E, Lin J-T, Mantey SA, Coy DH, Jensen RT (1992) Activation of neuromedin B-preferring bombesin receptors on rat glioblastoma C-6 cells alters cellular calcium and phosphoinositides. Biochem J (in press)

Westendorf JM, Schonbrunn A (1983) Characterization of bombesin receptors in a rat pituitary cell line. J Biol Chem 258:7527–7535

Willey JC, Lechner JF, Harris CC (1984) Bombesin and C-terminal tetradecapeptide of gastrin-releasing peptide are growth factors for normal human bronchial epithelial cells. Exp Cell Res 153:245–248

Woll PJ, Rozengurt E (1988) [D-Arg^1-,D-Phe^5,D-Trp^{7,9},Leu^{11}]-substance P: a potent bombesin antagonist in murine Swiss 3T3 cells inhibits the growth of human small-cell lung cancer cells in vitro. Proc Natl Acad Sci USA 85:1859–1863

Woll PJ, Coy DH, Rozengurt E (1988) [Leu^{13}-psi(CH_2NH)Leu^{14}]bombesin is a specific bombesin receptor antagonist in Swiss 3T3 cells. Biochem Biophys Res Commun 155:359–365

Yachnis AT, Crawley JN, Jensen RT, McGrane HM, Moody TW (1984) The antagonism of bombesin in the CNS by substance P analogues. Life Sci 35:1963–1969

Zachary I, Rozengurt E (1985) High affinity receptors for peptides of the bombesin family in Swiss 3T3 cells. Proc Natl Acad Sci USA 82:7616–7620

Zhang L, Mantey S, Jensen RT, Gardner JD (1988) An analogue of substance P with broad receptor antagonist activity. Biochim Biophys Acta 972:37–44

Bombesin Antagonists: Experimental and Clinical Results

J. Schütte and S. Seeber

Innere Klinik und Poliklinik (Tumorforschung), Westdeutsches Tumorzentrum, Universitätsklinikum Essen, Hufelandstraße 55, W-4300 Essen 1, FRG

Introduction

Lung cancer is the leading cause of cancer deaths in North America and Western Europe. Despite considerable knowledge of the genetic changes involving protooncogenes and tumor suppressor genes in lung cancer pathogenesis, and significant therapeutic progress achieved during the early 1980s with use of radio- and chemotherapy, overall treatment outcome remains poor for most patients. To design alternative therapeutic strategies in this disease, it is important to work toward the identification of mitogenic factors and a more complete understanding of the signal transduction pathways that stimulate lung cancer cell growth.

Small-cell lung cancer (SCLC), which constitutes about 25% of bronchogenic carcinomas, as well as pulmonary carcinoids and a small fraction of non-small-cell lung cancers are characterized by the presence of intracytoplas-

Table 1. Autocrine and paracrine growth factors for small-cell lung cancer and pulmonary carcinoid cells

Growth factor	Autocrine	Paracrine
Gastrin-releasing peptide/bombesin	+	
Neuromedin B	+	
Neuromedin C	+	
Ranatensin	+	
Litorin	+	
Neurotensin	+	
Vasopressin	+	
Cholecystokinin	+	
Serotonin	+	
Insulin-like growth factor I	+	
Galanin	+	+
Bradykinin		+
Acetylcholine		+

Recent Results in Cancer Research, Vol. 129

mic neurosecretory granules and by the ability to secrete many hormones and neuropeptides, including bombesin, neuromedin B, neurotensin, cholecystokinin, and vasopressin (Bepler et al. 1988a; Carney et al. 1985; Giaccone et al. 1992; Korman et al. 1986; Luster et al. 1985; Moody et al. 1991; Sausville et al. 1986; Sethi and Rozengurt 1991a; Sethi et al. 1992; Wood et al. 1981). It has been shown that many of these neuropeptides regulate growth of SCLC in an autocrine or paracrine fashion (Table 1). Among the best studied autocrine growth factors in SCLC is the gastrin-releasing peptide (GRP) which is thought to represent the mammalian homologue of the amphibian peptide bombesin (Battey et al. 1991; Lebacq-Verheyden et al. 1988; Sausville et al. 1986; Spindel et al. 1984).

Structure and Function of Bombesin/GRP

Structure and Tissue Expression of Bombesin/GRP

Bombesin is a 14-amino acid peptide initially isolated from the skin of two European frogs, *Bombina bombina* and *Bombina veriegata veriegata* (Anastasi 1971). In amphibians, the bombesin-like peptides are classified into three subfamilies: the bombesins, the ranatensins, and the phyllolitorins (Table 2). The family of bombesin-like neuropeptides includes GRP, neuromedin C, and alytesin. In mammals, neuropeptides of the bombesin family are produced by neurons of the central and peripheral nervous system and by normal cells of the dispersed neuroendocrine system, such as pulmonary neuroendocrine (PNE) cells (Brown et al. 1978; Dockray et al. 1979; McDonald et al. 1978; Tache and Brown 1982; Wharton et al. 1978).

Table 2. Amino acid sequences of bombesin/GRP, substance P, and analogues

Bombesins	
GRP	Val-Pro-Leu-Pro-Ala-Gly-Gly-Gly-Thr-Val-Leu-Thr-Lys- -Met-Tyr-Pro-Arg-Gly-Asn-His-**Trp**-**Ala**-Val-**Gly**-His-*Leu*-**Met**-**NH$_2$**
Bombesin	pGlu-Gln-Arg-Leu-Gly-Asn-Gln-**Trp**-**Ala**-Val-**Gly**-His-*Leu*-**Met**-**NH$_2$**
Ranatensins	
Neuromedin B	Gly-Asn-Leu-**Trp**-**Ala**-Thr-**Gly**-His-Phe-**Met**-**NH$_2$**
Ranatensin	pGlu-Val-Pro-Gln-**Trp**-**Ala**-Val-**Gly**-His-Phe-**Met**-**NH$_2$**
Litorin	pGlu-Gln-**Trp**-**Ala**-Val-**Gly**-His-Phe-**Met**-**NH$_2$**
Phyllolitorins	
Leu-8 Phyllolitorin	pGlu-Leu-**Trp**-**Ala**-Val-**Gly**-Ser-*Leu*-**Met**-**NH$_2$**
Tachykinins	
Neurokinin A	His-Lys-Thr-Asp-Ser-Phe-Val-Gly-*Leu*-**Met**-**NH$_2$**
Substance P	Arg-Pro-Lys-Pro-Gln-Gln-Phe-Phe-Gly-*Leu*-**Met**-**NH$_2$**
Antagonist A	DArg-DPro-Lys-Pro-Gln-Gln-DTrp-Phe-DTrp-*Leu*-Leu-**NH$_2$**
Antagonist D	DArg-Pro-Lys-Pro-DPhe-Gln-DTrp-Phe-DTrp-*Leu*-Leu-**NH$_2$**
Antagonist G	Arg-DTrp-MePhe-DTrp-*Leu*-Leu-**NH$_2$**

GRP, the mammalian homologue of bombesin, is a 27 amino acid peptide. It is formed by posttranslational processing of the prepro-GRP peptide involving several proteolytic cleavages and giving rise to GRP_{1-27}, GRP_{18-27} (neuromedin C), and GRP-gene associated peptides (G-GAPs) (Lebacq-Verheyden et al. 1988; Quinn et al. 1991; Spindel et al. 1984). The 14 amino acid carboxyl terminus of mammalian GRP shares significant homology with bombesin, and is thought to be responsible for receptor binding and biologic activity (Table 2). The sequence identity of the carboxyl-terminal heptapeptide between bombesin and GRP results in common antigens, as demonstrated by immune cross-reactivity of respective polyclonal antisera. Thus, GRP has been referred to as having bombesin-like immunoreactivity (BLI) which is predominantly found in brain, intestine, and fetal PNE cells (Brown et al. 1978; Ghatei et al. 1982; McGregor et al. 1982; Moody and Pert 1979; Panula 1986; Polak et al. 1976; Wharton et al. 1978). While BLI is readily detected in fetal and newborn lung, significant levels are absent in adult lung suggesting that bombesin/GRP has an important role in fetal lung function and/or differentiation (Wharton et al. 1978). In the normal lung, secretion of GRP by PNE cells occurs in response to alterations in pulmonary oxygenation and stimulation of the nicotinic cholinergic receptor (Cutz et al. 1981; Schüller 1992). Multifocal PNE cell hyperplasia has been observed in a variety of chronic inflammatory lung disease, and rats with experimental asbestosis have elevated lung tissue levels of BLI late in the course of disease (Schüller 1992). In asymptomatic cigarette smokers, elevated levels of BLI/GRP have been reported to occur in the bronchoalveolar lavage fluid (Aguayo et al. 1992). BLI/GRP has been detected also in human tumors and tumor cell lines thought to be derived from neuroendocrine cells, such as SCLC, pulmonary carcinoids, and medullary carcinoma of the thyroid (Bepler et al. 1988a; Carney et al. 1985, 1987; Luster et al. 1985; Moody et al. 1981; Sausville et al. 1986; Tamai et al. 1983; Wood et al. 1981; Yamaguchi et al. 1984). Elevated serum levels of BLI/GRP have been described in SCLC patients with extensive disease. Non-small-cell lung cancers usually show no or only low levels of BLI and GRP expression (Bepler et al. 1988a; Giaccone et al. 1992; Korman et al. 1986; Luster et al. 1985).

Bombesin/GRP-Induced Signal Transduction Pathways

Lung cancer cells thought to be derived from PNE cell origin, such as SCLC cells, express and secrete significant levels of bombesin/GRP, and some of the SCLC cell lines express high-affinity bombesin/GRP receptors on their cell surface (Cuttita et al. 1985; Moody et al. 1981, 1987; Weber et al. 1985). The bombesin/GRP receptor has been shown to be a member of the G protein coupled receptor family (Dohlman et al. 1987; Erusalimsky et al. 1988; Kris et al. 1987; Sethi et al. 1992; Sinnet-Smith et al. 1990). A similar receptor type has been demonstrated for other neuropeptide mitogens, including neuromedin B, angiotensin, serotonin, substance K, and substance P (Seithi et al. 1992). Upon binding to its receptor, bombesin/GRP, like other neuropeptides secreted by

SCLC cells, induces a cascade of intracellular signal transduction pathways resulting in DNA synthesis and increase of cellular proliferation about 10–16 h later (Moody et al. 1981; Schüller et al. 1990; Sethi and Rozengurt 1991 a, b; Sethi et al. 1992; Trepel et al. 1988 b; Zachary et al. 1991).

Most of these intracellular signal transduction pathways (Fig. 1) have been studied in detail in Swiss 3T3 cells which are characterized by expression of high numbers of bombesin/GRP receptors and by their responsiveness to exogeneous bombesin/GRP (for review see Sethi et al. 1992). One of the earliest findings in Swiss 3T3 cells after binding of bombesin/GRP to its receptor is a rapid mobilization of Ca^{2+} from internal stores, leading to transient increase in the intracellular Ca^{2+} concentration. This results from phospholipase C (PLC)-mediated hydrolysis of phosphatidylinositol 4,5-bisphosphate (PIP_2) leading to an increase in inositol-1,4,5-trisphosphate. In addition, diacylglycerol (DAG) is generated by this process as well as by phosphatidylcholine hydrolysis. DAG acts as a second messenger in the activation of protein kinase C, which in turn results in protein phosphorylation, stimulation of Na^+, H^+, and K^+ ions across the cell membrane, leading to cytoplasmic alkalinization and increased intracellular $[K^+]$. In addition, bombesin/GRP, as well as vasopressin and endothelin have been shown to induce rapid stimulation of tyrosine phosphorylation of several substrates in quiescent 3T3 cells (Sanders et al. 1988). Furthermore, bombesin/GRP induces a release of arachidonic acid and prostaglandin E_2 into the culture medium. This suggests that bombesin/GRP receptors may be coupled to PLC activation through a putative G protein and to arachidonic acid release through phospholipase A_2.

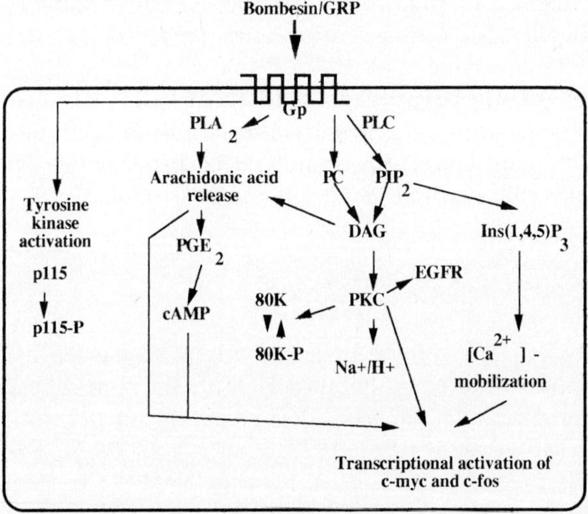

Fig. 1. Bombesin/GRP-induced signal transduction pathways in Swiss 3T3 cells. (Modified according to Sethi et al. 1992) (*Gp*, G protein; *PLA_2*, phospholipase A_2; *PLC*, phospholipase C; *PC*, phosphatidylcholine; *$Ins(1,4,5)P_3$*, inositol-(1,4,5)-trisphosphate; *DAG*, diacylglycerol; *PKC*, protein kinase C; *EGF-R*, epidermal growth factor receptor; *PIP_2* phosphatidylinositol-(1,4)-bisphosphate; *PGE_2*, prostaglandin E_2; *cAMP*, cyclic adenosine monophosphate)

Similar to oncogene activation by other growth factors, bombesin/GRP in Swiss 3T3 cells stimulates transient expression of the c-*fos* and c-*myc* protooncogenes (Cirillo et al. 1986; Moody et al. 1987; Schüller et al. 1990; Sethi and Rozengurt 1991 a, b; Sethie et al. 1992; Trepel et al. 1988 b; Zachary et al. 1991; for review see Sethi et al. 1992).

Some of the signal transduction pathways observed after incubation of Swiss 3T3 cells with bombesin/GRP have been confirmed in SCLC cells. This includes activation of PLC and increase in intracellular Ca^{2+} concentration. Interestingly, this effect was most pronounced in cell lines of so-called classical type (characterized by prominent neuroendocrine features including hormone production, relatively long doubling time) whereas 'variant type' SCLC cell lines (less or no expression of neuroendocrine markers, shorter doubling times, frequent c-*myc* amplification) were less sensitive to stimulation with bombesin/GRP (Carney et al. 1985; Heikkila et al. 1987; Moody et al. 1987; Sethi and Rozengurt 1991 a, b; Sethi et al. 1992; Trepel et al. 1988 a, b).

Mitogenic Effects of Bombesin/GRP on Lung Cancer Cells in Vitro and in Vivo

Bombesin/GRP stimulates in vitro proliferation of normal human bronchoepithelial cells (Willey et al. 1984). The effects of bombesin/GRP on the growth of lung cancer cells in vitro and in vivo have been extensively studied by numerous investigators. In several experiments, it was demonstrated that incubation of SCLC cells with exogenous bombesin/GRP stimulated their growth in liquid culture and clonal growth in soft agarose (Alexander et al. 1988; Bepler et al. 1988 a; Carney et al. 1987; Cuttita et al. 1985; Luster et al. 1985; Moody et al. 1981; Sethi and Rozengurt 1991 a, b; Sethi et al. 1992; Weber et al. 1985).

This effect was most pronounced when cells were incubated in serum-free defined medium. No significant differences were observed in the biologic effects of the original amphibian bombesin and the mammalian peptide GRP_{1-27}. Interestingly, stimulation of colony formation was not correlated with the expression of endogenous BLI or bombesin/GRP receptors (Carney et al. 1987). As an explanation of the latter observation, it has been hypothesized that growth-promoting effects of bombesin/GRP in these cell lines could be the result of mechanisms other than binding to specific receptors. Alternatively, only a small fraction of cells could possess receptors that would escape detection in the receptor assay. Finally, down-regulation of bombesin/GRP receptors, as observed in other cell types, could result from constant release of bombesin/GRP into the culture medium. In contrast to the observations made with SCLC, little or no stimulatory effect was observed in a panel of non-small-cell lung cancer cell lines which usually express only marginal or no BLI and bombesin/GRP receptors. Overall, these data demonstrate that bombesin/GRP has an important role in the in vitro growth of SCLC cells and suggest that in some instances bombesin/GRP may function as an autocrine growth factor.

In addition, in vivo proliferation of SCLC by bombesin/GRP has been described in experiments where the human SCLC cell line NCI-H69 was implanted into nude mice. Mice were randomized to be given bombesin or saline, and a significant increase of tumor weight over controls was observed 4–6 weeks later in those animals treated with bombesin (Alexander et al. 1988).

The most convincing evidence for an autocrine role of bombesin/GRP in SCLC is based on experiments by Cuttita et al. (1985). Using a monoclonal antibody (2A11) raised against a synthetic analogue of bombesin, they showed that this antibody could block the binding of bombesin/GRP to bombesin/GRP receptors in SCLC membrane preparations, and inhibit the clonal growth of two SCLC cell lines in vitro and the growth of SCLC xenografts in vivo.

Bombesin/GRP Antagonists

The data presented above have demonstrated that bombesin/GRP acts as an autocrine growth factor in a substantial number of SCLC cell lines in vitro and in vivo. In searching for new strategies to modulate SCLC growth in patients with this disease, several distinct mechanisms may be considered to disrupt the autocrine growth stimulation of SCLC cells by bombesin/GRP. First, synthetic analogues of bombesin/GRP could be used which occupy the receptor without activating signal transduction pathways by themselves, thus lacking agonist activity (for review see Jensen et al., "Bombesin receptor antagonists: different classes and cellular basis of action", this volume). Second, monoclonal antibodies such as 2A11 can be used to bind endogenous bombesin/GRP and block its binding to the receptor (Cuttita et al. 1985). Furthermore, bombesin/GRP is only one of several neuropeptides whose autocrine or paracrine growth stimulatory effects on SCLC cells involve similar or identical second messenger pathways. Thus, it is conceivable that disruption of pathways such as the intracellular Ca^{2+} mobilization, e.g., by use of calcium/calmodulin antagonists, will diminish the effects not only of bombesin/GRP but, simultaneously, of other peptides that stimulate SCLC proliferation (Schüller 1991, 1992; Schüller et al. 1990).

Synthetic Bombesin/GRP Antagonists

As described by Jensen et al. ("Bombesin receptor antagonists: different classes and cellular basis of action", this volume), a large number of synthetic bombesin analogues have been synthesized. Using Swiss 3T3 and pancreatic acinar cells as a test system in most analyses, some of these analogues exhibit significant bombesin/GRP antagonistic activity in vitro.

Substance P Analogues

So far, only a small number of analogues have undergone in vitro testing in SCLC cell lines. Initial synthetic antagonists analyzed in SCLC cells were analogues of substance P (Table 2). The first antagonist to be studied was [D-Arg^{1},D-Pro^{2},D-Trp^{7,9},Leu^{11}]substance P (antagonist A). Substance P is structurally unrelated to bombesin/GRP and has no bombesin/GRP antagonist activity; antagonist A was found to block the secretory effects of bombesin on a pancreatic preparation, diminish bombesin/GRP binding to its receptor and inhibit mitogenesis in Swiss 3T3 cells (Jensen et al. 1984; Zachary and Rozengurt 1986). However, it did not affect mitogenesis induced by polypeptide growth factors, such as platelet-derived growth factor and epidermal growth factor. In SCLC cell lines, [D-Arg^{1},D-Pro^{2},D-Trp^{7,9},Leu^{11}]substance P was described to inhibit the ability of bombesin/GRP to stimulate clonal growth of these cells and inhibit (^{3}H)thymidine incorporation of SCLC cells in liquid culture (Layton et al. 1988; Sethi et al. 1992; Woll and Rozengurt 1988, 1990; Zachary and Rozengurt 1986).

Among other congeners of substance P tested for bombesin/GRP antagonism, two compounds with inhibitory activity were identified: antagonist D, [D-Arg^{1},D-Phe^{5},D-Trp^{7,9}Leu^{11}]substance P, and antagonist G, [Arg^{6},D-Trp^{7,9},MePhe^{8}]substance P(6-11). Antagonist D was shown to be fivefold more potent than antagonist A in preventing the cellular effects of bombesin/GRP and vasopressin in mouse 3T3 cells and in inhibiting the growth of SCLC cells in serum-free medium. Overall, in Swiss 3T3 cells both antagonists were demonstrated to have in common the ability not only to inhibit the effects of bombesin/GRP but also the effects of other neuropeptides, including vasopressin, bradykinin, endothelin, and substance P. This is also reflected by data showing that antagonist G is tenfold less potent than antagonist D in blocking bombesin/GRP mediated mitogenesis in Swiss 3T3 cells it is almost as potent as antagonist D in inhibiting SCLC proliferation in vitro. In addition, antagonist G showed inhibition of SCLC xenografts in vivo (Sethi et al. 1992; Woll and Rozengurt 1988, 1990).

Together, the above data suggest that some effects of substance P antagonists may be due to inhibition of neuropeptides other than bombesin/GRP. Therefore, Rozengurt et al. have referred to these substances as broad-spectrum-antagonists (Sethi et al. 1992). The theoretical advantage of broad-spectrum activity, however, could be problematic when using these drugs in vivo because activity of several neuropeptides important for normal body function, including vasopressin and substance P itself, may be disrupted. In addition, substance P antagonists show antagonistic activity only in the micromolar range as opposed to the submicromolar doses required for newer compounds of different chemical structure (Bepler et al. 1988 b).

Reduced Peptide Bond Analogues of Bombesin. The synthetic peptide [Leu^{14}, ψ-CH_2NH-Leu^{14}]bombesin ([$\psi^{13,14}$,Leu^{14}]bombesin; where ψ indicates "cyclic") belongs to the class of bombesin analogues with a reduced peptide bond (Coy et al. 1991; and see Jensen et al., this volume, for review). Several studies using Swiss 3T3 and pancreatic acinar cells have demonstrated [Leu^{14},ψ-CH_2NH-Leu^{14}]bombesin to be about 50 times more potent than substance P analogues, with antagonist activity in the submicromolar range. [Leu^{14},ψ-CH_2NH-Leu^{14}]bombesin has been tested in SCLC cells in vitro and in vivo (Mahmoud et al. 1991; Trepel et al. 1988a). In SCLC cell line NCI-H345, Trepel et al. (1988a) analyzed the effects of this peptide on bombesin-stimulated PLC activity and intracellular Ca^{2+} mobilization. They found that [Leu^{14},ψ-CH_2NH-Leu^{14}]bombesin effectively blocked bombesin-induced accumulation of inositol(1,4,5)trisphosphate with an IC_{50} of 50 n*M*. The IC_{50} for inhibition of intracellular Ca^{2+} release by 100 n*M* bombesin was approximately 2.5 µ*M*. In addition, they tested the inhibition of clonal growth of NCI-H345 by [Leu^{14},ψ-CH_2NH-Leu^{14}]bombesin in defined serum-free medium. Significant growth inhibition occurred at concentrations $\geq$100 n*M*. Mahmoud et al. (1991) extended the analysis of [Leu^{14},ψ-CH_2NH-Leu^{14}]bombesin in SCLC cells. They found significant inhibition of clonal growth of some SCLC cell lines in the absence or presence of exogenously added bombesin at [Leu^{14},ψ-CH_2NH-Leu^{14}]bombesin concentrations $\geq$50 n*M*. In contrast, [Leu^{14},ψ-CH_2NH-Leu^{14}]bombesin was ineffective in two lung cancer cell lines (NCI-H520 and NCI-H727) expressing epidermal growth factor but not bombesin/GRP receptors. In addition, the in vivo ability of [Leu^{14},ψ-CH_2NH-Leu^{14}]bombesin to antagonize the growth of SCLC was investigated. Growth of SCLC cell line xenografts in nude mice was retarded by approximately 50% during weeks 3–5 after tumor cell implantation. In contrast, [D-Arg^1,D-Pro^2,D-$Trp^{7,9}$,Leu^{11}]substance P did not show significant inhibition of tumor formation at week 5.

In the latter study (Mahmoud et al. 1991), additional bombesin analogues were analyzed including [D-Nal^6,$\psi^{13,14}$,Phe^{14}]$bombesin^{6-14}$, and [Pyr^6, Phe^{13},$\psi^{13,14}$,Leu^{14}]$bombesin^{6-14}$. In assays of ^{125}I-GRP binding to SCLC cell line NCI-H345, [D-Nal^6,$\psi^{13,14}$,Phe^{14}]$bombesin^{6-14}$ was found to be about six times more potent than [Leu^{14},ψ-CH_2NH-Leu^{14}]bombesin, whereas [Pyr^6,Phe^{13},$\psi^{13,14}$,Leu^{14}]$bombesin^{6-14}$ was approximately as active as [Leu^{14},ψ-CH_2NH-Leu^{14}]bombesin. Both analogues as well as [D-Arg^1, D-Pro^2,D-$Trp^{7,9}$,Leu^{11}]substance P inhibited intracellular Ca^{2+} release and clonal growth of SCLC cell lines in vitro. However, in vivo inhibition of SCLC xenograft growth in nude mice was only about 20% for both [D-Nal^6,$\psi^{13,14}$,Phe^{14}]$bombesin^{6-14}$ and [Pyr^6,Phe^{13},$\psi^{13,14}$,Leu^{14}]$bombesin^{6-14}$ as compared to 50% inhibition observed with [Leu^{14},ψ-CH_2NH-Leu^{14}]bombesin (see above). The difference between in vitro and in vivo results, observed in particular with [D-Nal^6,$\psi^{13,14}$,Phe^{14}]$bombesin^{6-14}$, was explained by a possibly higher degradation of the latter compound by endogenous proteases as compared to [Leu^{14},ψ-CH_2NH-Leu^{14}]bombesin. In summary, these data clearly demonstrate the need for in vivo testing of new analogues.

Monoclonal Antibodies

A murine monoclonal antibody (2A11) was developed by Cuttita et al. (1985) against a synthetic analogue of bombesin (Lys 3-bombesin). This antibody was shown to bind to GRP_{1-27}, GRP_{14-27}, and GRP_{20-27} but exhibited only insignificant or no binding to GRP_{22-27}, GRP_{1-16}, or substance P, or other tachykinins. It readily detected bombesin/GRP immunoreactivity in extracts of a series of SCLC cell lines but not of non-small-cell lung cancer cell lines and did not bind to live, intact SCLC. As 2A11 binds to the C-terminal region of GRP, it was tested for its ability to block the binding of labeled bombesin to its cell-surface receptor on SCLC cells. In fact, it was found to block the bombesin-receptor interaction in a dose-dependent fashion and almost completely inhibited bombesin binding at 10 n*M*. When tested in vitro, this antibody showed significant inhibition of clonal growth of two SCLC cell lines both of which produce detectable levels of bombesin/GRP. In nude mice xenograft studies, 2A11 significantly inhibited tumor formation in two of five mice treated intraperitoneally three times weekly. Tumors of control animals initially subjected to phosphate-buffered saline administration upon treatment with 2A11 stopped growing and became necrotic.

Pharmacokinetic studies of 2A11 in normal BALB/c mice demonstrated an initial clearance half-life of 24 h and a secondary clerance half-life of 1039 h (Avis et al. 1991). Biodistribution analysis revealed a distribution pattern which generally reflected blood flow. Toxicology studies in normal dogs (with gastric fistulas for gastric acid output analysis) infused with 50 mg 2A11 intravenously three times a week for 4 weeks failed to reveal any adverse behavioral, clinical, or pathological effects. Four of six dogs developed an immune response to 2A11. While anti-idiotypic antibodies elicited in two dogs did not mimic the functional effects of GRP, the emergence of an anti-mouse immunoglobulin response radically decreased half-life of 2A11 and compromised effective inhibition of bombesin/GRP-mediated biologic effects. It has been suggested that some of these immune responses could have been due to impurities of 2A11 preparations and may be prevented with a more purified 2A11 preparation (Avis et al. 1991).

In a clinical phase I study including 14 patients with advanced, previously treated lung cancer, 2A11 toxicity was analyzed (Mulshine et al. 1990). Four dose levels (1, 10, 100, 250 mg/m^2) were evaluated using a three times per week for 4 weeks delivery schedule. No clinical toxicity was reported. In particular, no patient had therapy discontinued due to immune responses to mouse immunoglobulin, and no or only modest changes in 2A11 clearance were observed. Based on a mathematical model to predict the requisite amount of antibody to neutralize growth factor (GRP) effect, it was suggested that for a future phase II trial 2A11 doses on the order of 200 mg per injection should be sufficient to block GRP effects in vivo (Mulshine et al. 1992).

Second Messenger Inhibition

As the intracellular effects of a number of neuropeptides produced by SCLC cells, including bombesin/GRP, are mediated at least in part through Ca^{2+} and calmodulin-dependent second messenger pathways, it has been proposed that action of these neuropeptides could be blocked by calcium/calmodulin antagonists. An impressive animal model system to study this hypothesis has been developed by Schüller et al. (1990). Using Syrian golden hamsters maintained under hyperoxic conditions and treatment with carcinogenic *N*-nitrosodiethylamine (DEN) as cancer-inducing chemical, animals reproducibly develop neuroendocrine lung tumors. These tumors demonstrate high levels of immunoreactivity to mammalian bombesin and calcitonin. Tumor cells also express acetylcholine receptors of the nicotine type which have been shown to regulate tumor cell secretion of bombesin/GRP. Both the nicotine receptor and the bombesin/GRP receptor operate at least in part via ion channels with a high affinity for Ca^{2+} as second messenger (Hucho 1986; Sethi and Rozengurt 1991 a). The signal transduction pathway utilizes calmodulin further downstream for the processing of intracellular Ca^{2+}.

Based on these and other data (Gietzen et al. 1990; Sanders set al. 1988; Schüller et al. 1991; Überall et al. 1991) showing that B859-35, a (–)enantiomer of the dihydropyridine derivative niguldipine which lacks clinically significant antihypertensive activity, has antiproliferative activity on the neuroendocrine lung cancer cell line NCI-H727 (a carcinoid cell line) in vitro, Schüller et al. (1990) used B859-35 to test its ability to suppress lung tumor formation in a hamster animal model. Interestingly, a significant anticarcinogenic effect of B859-35 was observed on the formation of neuroendocrine lung tumors and nasal cavity tumors in those animals which were given B859-35 intragastrically 5 days per week for 20 weeks. Neuroendocrine lung tumors were observed in 62% of control animals treated with DEN and hyperoxia, and in none of 12 animals receiving DEN and hyperoxia plus B859-35. It has been suggested that this effect may be due to the inhibition of Ca^{2+}/calmodulin and proteinkinase C by B859-35. Whether a similar impressive antiproliferative effect of B859-35 can be observed in human SCLC, which is usually less well-differentiated than the carcinoid cell line NCI-H727 and the hamster neuroendocrine lung tumors, remains to be proven by further in vitro studies and currently conducted clinical trials.

Conclusions

With the discovery that SCLC growth is regulated by a number of paracrine and autocrine growth factors such as bombesin/GRP, some interesting new concepts with potential clinical relevance have been developed over the past several years. In the case of bombesin/GRP, these include the development of synthetic bombesin/GRP antagonists, monoclonal antibodies directed against the receptor-binding domain of bombesin/GRP, and use of drugs that might interfere with second messenger pathways used by bombesin/GRP as well as other neuropeptides relevant for SCLC proliferation. As shown above, all three concepts have yielded promising initial results in vitro and in vivo.

Prior to including these concepts into clinical treatment strategies, however, a number of questions remain to be answered. First, interactions of mitogenic neuropeptides and their receptors in SCLC are not yet entirely unraveled. As an example, it has recently been shown that neuromedin B and its receptor which share significant homology with GRP and the GRP receptor, respectively, are expressed in many SCLC cell lines (Giaccone et al. 1992; Krane et al. 1988; Wada et al. 1990, 1991). Since neuromedin B can stimulate SCLC growth in vitro (Bepler et al. 1988 a), this suggests that neuromedin B could act as an autocrine growth factor. In addition, both GRP and neuromedin B can bind to each other's receptor although with different affinities (Wada et al. 1991). Thus, it is conceivable that, despite efficient high-specificity inhibition of GRP receptors by synthetic analogues or monoclonal antibodies, GRP and neuromedin B may continue to stimulate SCLC cell proliferation via neuromedin B receptors. On the other hand, as bombesin/GRP is a neurotransmitter regulating the secretion of several gastrointestinal and pituitary hormones, it remains to be shown if plasma levels of synthetic antagonists required to efficiently block both receptors may eventually produce significant clinical toxicity.

A theoretical advantage for using synthetic peptides instead of monoclonal antibodies such as 2A11 would be their proposed higher penetration into tumor tissue. In addition, immune responses to murine immunoglobulins may alter antibody half-life and compromise its growth inhibitory effects, as observed in animal studies (Avis et al. 1991). On the other hand, monoclonal antibodies such as 2A11 will not or only marginally cross the blood-brain barrier, and this characteristic has been suggested to have contributed to its lack of clinically significant toxicity in a recent phase I trial (Avis et al. 1991; Mulshine et al. 1990, 1992).

Broad-spectrum signal transduction antagonists such as the dihydropyridine derivative B859-35 which interfere with Ca^{2+}/calmodulin and protein kinase C-mediated second messenger pathways are attractive compounds with potential antiproliferative activity in SCLC. However, as the signal transduction pathways induced by bombesin/GRP, neuromedin B, and other autocrine or paracrine growth factors operative in SCLC are not entirely known, it remains speculative if such agents will be able to effectively block intracellular growth factor action responsible for proliferation of these cells in vivo.

Overall, the results obtained so far from in vitro and in vivo (animal) experiments with synthetic bombesin/GRP analogues, monoclonal antibodies and second messenger antagonists such as B859-35 are encouraging in terms of their possible use as anticancer agents in SCLC. Further phase I clinical trials are warranted to carefully elucidate their pharmacokinetics and their toxicity including possible immune respones. It is conceivable that such agents if showing no or moderate toxicity could be used as an adjunct to conventional chemo-/radiotherapy in induction therapy, and/or as adjuvant treatment after achieving complete remission with the latter treatment modalities.

References

Aguayo SM, King TE, Kane MA, Sherritt KM, Silvers W, Nett LM, Petty TL, Miller YE (1992) Urinary levels of bombesin-like peptides in asymptomatic cigarette smokers: a potential risk marker for smoking-related diseases. Cancer Res [Suppl] 52:2727s–2731s

Alexander RW, Upp JR, Poston GJ, Gupta V, Townsend CM, Thompson JC (1988) Effects of bombesin on growth of human small cell lung carcinoma in vivo. Cancer Res 48:1439–1441

Anastasi A, Erspamer V, Bucci M (1971) Isolation and structure of bombesin alytesin, two analogous active peptides from the skin of the European amphibians Bombina and Alytes. Experientia 27:166–167

Avis IL, Kovacs TOG, Kasprzyk PG, Treston AM, Bartholonew R, Walsh JH, Cuttita F, Mulshine JL (1991) Preclinical evaluation of an anti-autocrine growth factor monoclonal antibody for treatment of patients with small-cell lung cancer. J Natl Cancer Inst 83:1470–1476

Battey JF, Way JM, Corjay MH, Shapira H, Kusano K, Harkins R, Wu JM, Slattery T, Mann E, Feldmann RI (1991) Molecular cloning of the bombesin/gastrin-releasing peptide receptor from Swiss 3T3 cells. Proc Natl Acad Sci USA 88:395–399

Bepler G, Rotsch M, Jaques G, Haeder M, Heymanns J, Hartogh G, Kiefer P, Havemann K (1988a) Peptides and growth factors in small cell lung cancer: production, binding sites, and growth effects. J Cancer Res Clin Oncol 114:235–244

Bepler G, Zeymer U, Mahmoud S, Fiskum G, Palszynski E, Rotsch M, Willey J, Koros A, Cuttita F, Moody TW (1988b) Substance P analogues function as bombesin receptor antagonists and inhibit small cell lung cancer clonal growth. Peptides 9:1367–1372

Brown M, Allen R, Villareal J, Rivier J, Vale W (1978) Bombesin-like activity: radioimmunologic assessment in biological tissues. Life Sci 23:2721–2726

Carney DN, Gazdar AF, Bepler G, Guccion JG, Marangos PJ, Moody TW, Zweig MH, Minna JD (1985) Establishment and identification of small cell lung cancer cell lines having classical and variant features. Cancer Res 45:2913–2923

Carney DN, Cuttita F, Moody TW, Minna JD (1987) Selective stimulation of small cell lung cancer clonal growth by bombesin and gastrin-related peptide. Cancer Res 47:821–825

Cirillo DM, Gaudino G, Naldini L, Comoglio PM (1986) Receptor for bombesin with associated tyrosine kinase activity. Mol Cell Biol 6:4641–4649

Coy DH, Jiang NY, Kim SH, Moreau JP, Lin JT, Frucht H, Qian JM, Wang LW, Jensen RT (1991) Covalently cyclized agonist and antagonist analogues of bombesin and related peptides. J Biol Chem 266:16441–16447

Cuttita F, Carney DN, Mulshine J, Moody TW, Fedorko J, Fischler A, Minna JD (1985) Bombesin-like peptides can function as autocrine growth factors in human small-cell lung cancer. Nature 316:823–826

Cutz E, Chan W, Track NS (1981) Bombesin, calcitonin, and leukenkaphalin immunoreactivity in endocrine cells of human lung. Experientia 37:765–767

Dockray GJ, Vaillant C, Walsh JH (1979) The neuronal origin of bombesin-like immunoreactivity in the rat gastrointestinal tract. Neuroscience 4:1561–1568

Dohlman HG, Caron MG, Lefkowitz RJ (1987) A family of receptors coupled to guanine nucleotide regulatory proteins. Biochem J 26:2657–2664

Erusalimsky JD, Friedberg I, Rozengurt E (1988) Bombesin, diacylglycerols and phorbol esters rapidly stimulate the phosphorylation of an M_r 80000 protein kinase C substrate in permeabilized 3T3 cells: effect of guanine nucleotides. J Biol Chem 263:19188–19194

Ghatei MA, Jung RT, Stevenson JC, Hiiyard CJ, Adrian TC, Lee YC, Christofides ND, Sarson DL, Nashiter K, MacIntyre I, Bloom SR (1982) Bombesin action on gut hormones and calcium in man. J Clin Endocrinol Metab 54:980–985

Giaccone G, Battey J, Gazdar AF, Oie H, Draoui M, Moody TW (1992) Neuromedin B is present in lung cancer cell lines. Cancer Res [Suppl] 52:2732s–2736s

Gietzen K, Bai G, Abdallah F (1990) Selective inhibition of proliferation by a novel dihydropyridine derivative with anti-calmodulin activitiy in the mammary tumour cell line ZR-75-1. Med Sci Res 18:627–629

Heikkila R, Trepel JB, Cuttita F, Neckers LM, Sausville R (1987) Bombesin-related peptides induce calcium mobilization in a subset of human small cell lung cancer cell lines. J Biol Chem 262:16456–16460

Hucho F (1986) The nicotinic acetylcholine receptor and its ion channels. Eur J Biochem 158:211–226

Jensen RT, Jones SW, Folkers K, Gardner JD (1984) A synthetic peptide that is a bombesin receptor antagonist. Nature 309:61–63

Korman LY, Carney DN, Citron ML, Moody TW (1986) Secretin/vasoactive peptide-stimulated secretion of bombesin/gastrin releasing peptide from human small cell carcinoma of the lung. Cancer Res 46:1214–1218

Krane IM, Naylor SL, Helin-Davis D, Chin WW, Spindel ER (1988) Molecular cloning of cDNAs encoding the human bombesin-like peptide neuromedin B. J Biol Chem 263:13317–13323

Kris RM, Hazan R, Villines J, Moody TW, Schlessinger J (1987) Identification of the bombesin receptor on murine and human cells by cross-linking experiments. J Biol Chem 262:11215–11220

Layton JE, Scanlon DB, Soveny C, Morstyn G (1988) Effects of bombesin antagonists on the growth of small cell lung cancer cells in vitro. Cancer Res 48:4783–4789

Lebacq-Verheyden AM, Kaprzyk PG, Raum MG, Van Wyke Coelingh K, Lebacq JA, Battey JF (1988) Posttranslational processing of endogenous and baculovirus-expressed human gastrin releasing peptide precursor. Mol Cell Biol 8:3129–3135

Luster W, Gropp C, Kern HF, Havemann K (1985) Lung tumor cell lines synthesizing peptide hormones established from tumours of four histological types: characterization of the cell lines and analysis of their peptide hormone production. Br J Cancer 51:865–875

Mahmoud S, Staley J, Taylor J, Bogden A, Moreau JP, Coy D, Avis I, Cuttita F, Mulshine JL, Moody TW (1991) [Psi^{13,14},Leu^{14}]bombesin analogues inhibit growth of small cell lung cancer in vitro and in vivo. Cancer Res 51:1798–1802

McDonald TJ, Nilsson G, Vagne M, Ghatei M, Bloom SR, Mutt V (1978) A gastrin releasing peptide from the porcine non-antral gastric tissue. Gut 19:767–774

McGregor GP, Woodhams PL, O'Shaugnessy D, Ghatei MA, Polak JM, Bloom SR (1982) Developmental changes in bombesin, substance P, somatostatin, and vasoactive intestinal polypeptide in rat brain. Neurosci Lett 28:21–27

Moody TW, Pert CB (1979) Bombesin-like peptides in rat brain. Biochem Biophys Res Commun 90:7–14

Moody TW, Pert CB, Gazdar AF, Carney DN, Minna JD (1981) High levels of intracellular bombesin characterize human small-cell lung carcinoma. Science 214:1246–1248

Moody TW, Murphy A, Mahmoud S, Fiskum G (1987) Bombesin-like peptides elevate cytosolic calcium in small cell lung cancer cells. Biochem Biophys Res Commun 147:189–195

Mulshine J, Avis I, Carrasquillo J, Merchant B, Boland C, Perentesis P, Reynolds J, Larson S, Treston A, Scott F, Kasprzyk P, Johnson B, Ihde D, Gazdar A, Cuttita F, Minna JD (1990) Phase I study of an anti gastrin releasing peptide (GRP) monoclonal antibody in patients with lung cancer. Proc Am Assoc Clin Oncol 9:230 (abstr)

Mulshine JL, Shuke N, Daghighian F, Carrasquillo J, Ghosh B, Walsh T, Avis I, Reynolds R, Cuttita F, Larson SM (1992) The correct dose: pharmacologically guided end point for anti-growth factor therapy. Cancer Res [Suppl] 52:2743s–2746s

Panula P (1986) Histochemistry and function of bombesin-like peptides. Med Biol 64:177–192

Polak JM, Bloom SR, Hobbs S, Solcia E, Pearse AGE (1976) Distribution of bombesin-like peptide in human gastrointestinal tract. Lancet I:1109–1110

Quinn KA, Treston AM, Scott FM, Kaprzyk PG, Avis I, Siegfried JM, Mulshine JL, Cuttita F (1991) Alpha-amidation of peptide hormones in lung cancer. Cancer Cells 3:504–510

Sanders KH, Boer R, Eltze M, Galvan J (1988) Differential vascular and cardiac effects of the enantiomers of three dihydropyridine calcium antagonists, niguldipine, nitrendipine, and felodipine. Arch Pharmacol 338 [Suppl]:R36

Sausville EA, Lebacq-Verheyden AM, Spindel ER, Cuttita F, Gazdar AF, Battey JF (1986) Expression of the gastrin-releasing peptide gene in human small cell lung cancer. J Biol Chem 261:2451–2457

Schüller HM (1991) Receptor-mediated mitogenesis signals and lung cancer. Cancer Cells 3:496–503

Schüller HM (1992) Nitrosamine-induced lung carcinogenesis and Ca^{2+}/calmodulin antagonists. Cancer Res [Suppl] 52:2723s–2726s

Schüller HM, Correa E, Orloff M, Reznik GK (1990) Successful chemotherapy of experimental neuroendocrine lung tumors in hamsters with an antagonist of Ca^{2+}/calmodulin. Cancer Res 50:1645–1649

Schüller HM, Orloff M, Reznik GK (1991) Antiproliferative effects of the Ca^{2+}/calmodulin antagonist B859-35 and the Ca^{2+}/channel blocker verapamil on human lung cancer cell lines. Carcinogenesis 12:2301–2303

Sethi T, Rozengurt E (1991 a) Multiple neuropeptides stimulate clonal growth of small cell lung cancer: effects of bradykinin, vasopressin, cholecystokinin, galanin, and neurotensin. Cancer Res 51:3621–3623

Sethi T, Rozengurt E (1991 b) Galanin stimulates Ca^{2+} mobilization, inositol phosphate accumulation, and clonal growth in small cell lung cancer cells. Cancer Res 51:1674–1679

Sethi T, Langdon S, Smyth J, Rozengurt E (1992) Growth of small cell lung cancer cells: stimulation by multiple neuropeptides and inhibition by broad spectrum antagonists in vitro and in vivo. Cancer Res [Suppl] 52:2737s–2742s

Sinnet-Smith J, Lehmann W, Rozengurt E (1990) Bombesin receptor in membranes from Swiss 3T3 cells. Biochem J 265:485–493

Spindel ER, Chin WW, Price J, Rees LH, Besser GM, Habener JF (1984) Cloning and characterization of cDNAs encoding human gastrin-releasing peptide. Proc Natl Acad Sci USA 81:5699–5703

Tache Y, Brown M (1982) On the role of bombesin in homeostasis. Trends Neurosci 5:431–433

Tamai S, Kameya T, Yamafuchi K, Yanai N, Abe K, Yanaihara N, Yamazaki H, Kegeyama K (1983) Peripheral lung carcinoid tumor producing predominantly gastrin-releasing peptide (GRP). Cancer 52:273–281

Trepel JB, Moyer JD, Cuttita F, Frucht H, Coy DH, Natale RB, Mulshine JL, Jensen RT, Sausville EA (1988 a) A novel bombesin receptor antagonist inhibits autocrine signals in a small cell lung carcinoma cell line. Biochem Biophys Res Commun 156:1383–1389

Trepel JB, Moyer JD, Heikkila R, Sausville EA (1988 b) Modulation of bombesin-induced phosphatidylinositol hydrolysis in small-cell lung-cancer cell line. Biochem J 255:403–410

Überall F, Maly K, Egle A, Doppler W, Hofmann T, Grunicke HH (1991) Inhibition of cell proliferation, protein kinase C_1 and phorbolester-induced fos expression by the dihydropyridine derivative B859-35. Cancer Res 51:5821–5825

Wada E, Way J, Lebacq-Verheyden AM, Battey JF (1990) Neuromedin B and gastrin releasing peptide mRNAs are differentially distributed in the rat nervous system. J Neurosci 10:2917–2930

Wada E, Way J, Shapira H, Kusano K, Lebacq-Verheyden AM, Coy D, Jensen R, Battey J (1991) cDNA cloning, characterization and brain region-specific expression of a neuromedin-B preferring bombesin receptor. Neuron 6:421–430

Weber S, Zuckerman JE, Bostwick DG, Bensch KG, Sikic BI, Raffin TA (1985) Gastrin releasing peptide is a selective mitogen for small cell lung carcinoma in vitro. J Clin Invest 75:306–309

Wharton J, Polak JM, Bloom SR, Ghatei MA, Solcia E, Brown MR, Pearse AGE (1978) Bombesin-like immunoreactivity in the lung. Nature 273:769–770

Willey JC, Lechner JF, Harris CC (1984) Bombesin and the C-terminal tetradecapeptide of gastrin-releasing peptide are growth factors for normal human bronchial cells. Exp Cell Res 153:245–248

Woll PJ, Rozengurt E (1988) [D-Arg^{1},D-Phe^{5},D-$Trp^{7,9}$,Leu^{14}]substance P, a potent bombesin antagonist in murine Swiss 3T3 cells, inhibits the growth of human small cell lung cancer cells in vitro. Proc Natl Acad Sci USA 85:1859–1863

Woll PJ, Rozengurt E (1990) A neuropeptide antagonist that inhibits the growth of small cell lung cancer in vitro. Cancer Res 5:3968–3973

Wood SM, Wood JR, Ghatei MA, Lee YC, O'Shaughnessy D, Bloom SR (1981) Bombesin, somatostatin and neurotensin-like immunoreactivity in bronchial carcinoma. J Clin Endocrinol Metab 53:1310–1312

Yamaguchi K, Abe K, Adachi I, Suzuki M, Kimura S, Kameya T, Yanaihara N (1984) Concomitant production of immunoreactive gastrin-releasing peptide and calcitonin in medullary carcinoma of the thyroid. Metabolism 33:724–727

Zachary I, Rozengurt E (1986) A substance P antagonist also inhibits specific binding and mitogenic effects of vasopressin and bombesin-related peptides in Swiss 3T3 cells. Biochem Biophys Res Commun 137:135–141

Zachary I, Gil J, Lehmann W, Sinnet-Smith J, Rozengurt E (1991) Bombesin, vasopressin, and endothelin rapidly stimulate tyrosine phosphorylation in intact Swiss 3T3 cells. Proc Natl Acad Sci USA 88:4577–4581

Subject Index